"Drawing inspiration from the life and thought of Ludwig Wittgenstein, Haber's remarkable book offers a deeply illuminating exploration of language at the heart of psychoanalytic practice—what entices, what expands, and what forecloses, in our meaning-making endeavors. Elegantly weaving philosophy, clinical wisdom, and personal reflection, it celebrates the transformative power of dialogue and shared discovery. With intellectual generosity and emotional warmth, his work honors analysis as a creative, humane endeavor—one in which meaning, connection, and new possibilities emerge through courageous conversation—a 'syntax of coexistence' that is emancipatory."

William J. Coburn, *Founding Editor Emeritus,*
Psychoanalysis, Self and Context

"There are many evocative moments in the vignettes in Darren Haber's exciting new book. Both humane and intellectually rigorous, WORDS APART invites us to consider the implications of the intertwining of Wittgenstein's conception of the uses (and abuses) of language with the experience-near applications of intersubjectivity theory in clinical practice. Fear no bewitchment of the reader's intelligence, in this important exercise in psychotherapeutic understanding. Rather, take this as a recommendation of its bracing message for clinicians of all stripes."

Dennis Palumbo, *licensed psychotherapist and author*

"Darren Haber offers an eloquent 'first step in speaking of the confinement' inherent in the words and syntax we use, addressing the 'imperative need for creativity with words in pushing past the confining edges of clinical limits.' His book is a welcome complement to the growing emphasis on nonverbal process in psychoanalysis. Explicit words and implicit cues are not dichotomous processes; rather, they are integral dimensions of the 'talking cure.' Like interpretation itself, words remain essential, and Haber helps us think more deeply about the language we use and the impact it carries in our clinical work."

Dan Perlitz, *Supervising Psychoanalyst and Treasurer,*
International Association of Psychoanalytic Self Psychology

Dissociation, Compulsion, and Language Games in Psychoanalysis

Dissociation, Compulsion, and Language Games in Psychoanalysis investigates the strangely underexplored topic of the phenomenology of language in psychoanalytic dialogue—as impacted by trauma, addiction, and other compulsive aversions.

Drawing on the long tradition of phenomenology and exploration of the importance of language in philosophy, as well as the author's extensive clinical experience, this book explores how language acts as the interface of human connection and how, without really understanding what it is and how it functions, true communication and connection cannot be achieved. The author looks at how we can use the concept of family resemblance in the way we use words to come to an understanding of each other, so that even if we don't use language in exactly the same way, we can find common ground that let's us understand and empathize with each other.

With rich clinical vignettes and a fresh new application of philosophical ideas, this is key reading for all psychoanalysts and psychotherapists.

Darren Haber is a psychoanalyst practicing in West Los Angeles. He specializes in treating childhood trauma, addiction, and anxiety/depression. His book, *Circles Without a Center: Addiction, Accommodation and Vulnerability in Psychoanalysis*, was published in July 2022 by Routledge. He publishes a weekly Substack column called "Hearing the Worlds of Others" and is the winner of several analytic writing awards. He frequently teaches, and has published numerous papers in the journals *Psychoanalysis, Self and Context*, and *Psychoanalytic Inquiry*. His website is www.therapistinlosangeles.com. He is a senior member of the Institute of Contemporary Psychoanalysis and a member of the International Association for Psychoanalytic Self Psychology.

Dissociation, Compulsion, and Language Games in Psychoanalysis

Words Apart

Darren Haber

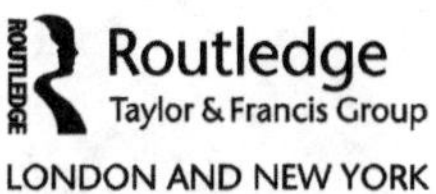

LONDON AND NEW YORK

First published 2027
by Routledge
4 Park Square, Milton Park, Abingdon, Oxon OX14 4RN

and by Routledge
605 Third Avenue, New York, NY 10158

Routledge is an imprint of the Taylor & Francis Group, an informa business

British Library Cataloguing-in-Publication Data
A catalogue record for this book is available from the British Library

ISBN: 978-1-032-98417-9 (hbk)
ISBN: 978-1-032-98061-4 (pbk)
ISBN: 978-1-003-59853-4 (ebk)

DOI: 10.4324/9781003598534

Typeset in Times New Roman
by codeMantra

This book is dedicated to Lucy and Elaine, whose support is invaluable … and to my patients, who teach me so much.

Contents

Preface

At the heart of our analytic investigations is a question, one that participants ask each other, and themselves: *What might this mean*? Patients speak, analysts respond, and meaning gradually emerges between two people, often surprised at the incompleteness of their understanding. This is especially true for patients whose optical prescriptions are outdated, for whom only the surface appears visible.

Making psychological sense seems to require a tolerance of opacity, as clinical conversation is a dialogue between histories, cultures, contexts, and *beliefs*, all supporting our way of using words and what we assume them to mean.

At times the capacity for misunderstanding seems so vast—a skyscraping Tower of Babel—that it is near-miraculous we understand one another at all.

Yet we also face, at one moment or another, the quiet terror of needing a listener, lest we speak into a void.

This book explores our dialogic processes through the philosophy of Ludwig Wittgenstein (2009) and his notion of *language games*.

So much depends upon shared agreements that ordinarily remain unnoticed. The background assumptions of our shared *forms of life*—Wittgenstein's (2009) description of language games—allow words to function as they do. Contrast can be disorienting when our patient, for instance, finds our focus on affect confusing, even threatening. Perhaps they know they are supposed to be talking about them, but cannot understand why.

Here participants might wonder about what is meant by "know," "understand," and the intent behind their use. Is knowing a theory, for instance, the same as knowing our patient? How do we come to understand them, and how do they imagine they understand us?

The point is that our acculturated understanding of terms and phrases, and their use, forms a *practice* rather than unassailable beliefs. Analysts assume that dreams carry symbolic meaning, that unconscious processes influence behavior, and that trauma can shape adaptation or provoke compulsive forms of numbing (mitigating painful forms of life).

But speaking of "trauma" can be disorienting for a newer patient. The volatility or neglect so profound to our ears is as common as the local weather.

The patient may ask what trauma *is*, and how it is treated. Will our explanations make sense?

So much depends upon cross-translation. The ragged process of "getting on the same page" reveals our nearly gothic interdependence.

What I am suggesting, in other words, is that psychological life is not so much described as *created* by our everyday language and theoretical practices, and their cross-pollination in analytic dialogue.

Language also maps our psychic forms of living. Not a stretch to say that, in some cases, patients' psychic meanings are not illuminated so much as *co-created* via dialogue, as with the meaning of dreams. The psychic map is also co-created, via cartographies of analytic exploration: those theories, communities, and personal histories shaping our perspective.

Such contexts, Wittgenstein (2009) believed, consist of what he called *grammar*: the background that makes our words intelligible.

Patients may speak of emotion in a grammatical jostling with the analyst's: as thing-like, a chess piece, perhaps unworthy of reflection. (Soon, we feel checkmated.) Affectivity, here, has not yet learned to talk. Strife may not register as calling for interpretation so much as spoiled produce ready for disposal.

Clinicians often refer to an *inner, psychic,* or *unconscious* process, but these too are framings, another kind of grammar repeatedly put into practice.

Determinate meanings arise through indeterminate processes. Understanding arrives not via static concepts but from the interactions and dialogue such concepts initiate. (Of course this, too, is a concept.) Often trouble arrives when one's cherished concepts cannot yield to revision, alternative views akin to a home invasion. A shadow struggle may break out between patient and analyst, where we want to plant a flag, insist that *this* is how it's done. Who gets to make the rules? (Such rules, Wittgenstein points out, are also contextually derived and "played," variable as dialects.)

Negotiation is constant. This too may be novel.

It is astonishing how our statements become heard outside of the speaker's intention. Often our intentions are opaque. When a weary patient says, "I did not get out of bed today," they may intend only that, as if the statement speaks for itself. Yet after much discussion, another meaning seeps out from between the gaps: a crushing despair, too heavy to discard or name, yet still not worth discussing. *What is there to talk about?* It is as if the patient's words will impact us as negatively as archaic criticism still grips their flexibilities of speech.

"I'm sorry to burden you with my depression," a patient once said to me. "I'm your *therapist*," I responded, "who else would you tell?"

Even more striking is the way in which difficulties are framed (e.g., as failure or weakness) which reveals an injured perspective that has never been allowed to speak. As a result the framing of a problem, for instance as an either/or, is most illustrative of the problem itself.

Treating addiction, as I often do, frequently begins with conflicting assumptions that are not immediately obvious. I emphasize psychological meaning; the patient measures progress in worldly or practical terms. My wanting to know more may be compassionate, intrusive, or a prompt for performance. "My bulimia has to do with my mother," a patient once said. I asked what made them say this. The answer: "Because my former therapist said so." And then silence.

The value of curiosity here may or may not register, landing as unfamiliarity for the patient rather than their "resistance." Our questions can *sound* simple, obvious—to us. Meanwhile what initially sounds hostile or dismissive from the patient may conceal an anxiety too shameful to acknowledge, perhaps regarding the difficulty of identifying affect. "It's like I lack the vocabulary," a highly intelligent patient once said of his emotionality, archaically disavowed in a volatile system.

It is often safer for all of us to cling to the familiar in a chaotically evolving world. Patients hold to well-worn binaries: *my family was fine; I am the problem; I disappoint everyone*. Such either/or narratives function as shelters, offering safety even as they isolate.

Yet these bunkers can be windowless, suffocating to expressivity. Relief is sought through compulsive activity such as drink, drugs, sex, or other means of soothing the strain of an undifferentiated life, so what is painful or *impossible* to say is no longer of concern. Dulled is the fraught dissatisfaction of unrecognized living, the sources of suffering rigidly elusive. (Some discuss everything except what brought them to treatment, and not only to distract.)

There is something quietly tragic in recognizing the untold devastation of patients' histories, how caregivers or societies have injured or neglected them. As patients begin to inhabit a more responsive relational space, past deprivations reveal themselves: fresh air contrasting the choking quality of smog.

My aim in this book is to examine how analytic dialogue unfolds when certainty reluctantly bends to curiosity—when both patient and analyst begin to question the assumptions that quietly organize their forms of life. I encourage readers to reflect upon their own "*a priori*" beliefs: the invisible background of certainties suddenly precarious in the heat of misunderstanding. I also hope to show how our expressions become bewitched, forms of life resistant to change (usually for self-protection). This can tempt us to provide a "counter-spell," when encountering rigidity, forgetting that new aspects of familiar vistas are not said but *shown,* via variances of perspective (which Wittgenstein [2009] calls shifts of aspect).

One of the enduring values of psychoanalysis, near sacred to this author, is a commitment to understanding—the stubborn effort to search for commonality, *family resemblances* of use (similar grammar): the cross-translations that make contact possible. At times it resembles the deciphering of signals from outer space.

The chapters that follow explore these questions through clinical moments, theoretical reflections, and philosophical influences. Rather than offering a unified doctrine, this book proceeds through a series of encounters—between analyst and patient, theory and experience, certainty and doubt. Each chapter examines a different way language shapes psychological life, and how analytic dialogue can loosen archaically rigid forms of silencing: the "rules" that govern how suffering is airbrushed as "selfish" or insignificant.

It may help to remember, in our contentious era, Wittgenstein's remark in his *Lecture on Ethics* (1993): that what is truly miraculous is not any particular statement *in* language but the very *existence* of language itself.

The same might be said of psychoanalysis. For all its difficulty, analytic dialogue allows two people to diligently co-create new forms of articulation—new forms of life—that enable patients to practice language games that possibly feel like home.

References

Wittgenstein, L. (2009). *Philosophical investigations* (4th ed.) (G.E.M. Anscombe, P.M.S. Hacker, & J. Schulte, Trans.) (P.M.S. Hacker, & J. Schulte, Eds.) Blackwell Publishing Ltd. Originally published 1953.

Wittgenstein, L. (1993). A lecture on ethics. In J. Klagge & A. Nordmann (Eds.), *Philosophical occasions 1912–1951* (pp. 37–44). Hackett Publishing Company.

Acknowledgments

Chapter 2, “Dissociation and Language Games in Psychoanalysis: Struck Dumb,” was originally published in *Psychoanalytic Inquiry*. Chapter 3, “Dissociation and Bewitchment in Analytic Dialogue: Having a Word,” was published in the online version of *The American Psychoanalyst*. Chapter 5, “Either/Or Language Games in Analytic Therapy: Yes or No,” was originally published in *Aeon Media Group Ltd.* The remaining chapters were originally published in abridged form via my Substack column, at darrenhaber.substack.com.

1 Introduction

Wittgenstein's Steam: Absence and Negotiation in Clinical Dialogue

Wittgenstein's Steam: Absence and Negotiation in Clinical Dialogue

Ludwig Wittgenstein lived on the edge of suicide for much of his life. What kept him alive was philosophy, specifically the need to understand language and what makes it comprehensible to us in the fluidity of everyday use. What counts as sensible or clear rather than confused or obscuring, according to what authority or standard?

Wittgenstein defined *language games* as contextually embedded *practices*, as "to imagine a language means to imagine a form of life" (2009, § 19). Our words are put into play against backgrounds as varied as tennis, charades, or video games—contexts (or systems) often taken for granted because we are embedded in them.

Wittgenstein's accent on words' *lived* significance leads Robert Stolorow to call him a "phenomenologist of language" (2020, personal communication). The context(s) of our use of words, practices of speech, leads to a defining syntax or *grammar* of our sentences (more on that below).

Psychoanalysis is often described as having its own inherited "rules" of play, according to community, custom, or idiosyncrasy—means of illuminating psychic "contents," unconscious meanings waiting to be recognized or brought into articulation. It is as if they were already somehow "there," under cover of the repressed, shunted aside via dissociation, or compulsively numbed—the latter suggesting a tangible "something" receiving a sedating I.V. drip.

This book presents a different view. Drawing on the philosophy of Ludwig Wittgenstein, I propose that analytic change does not primarily consist in *uncovering* preexisting meanings but in their gradual co-creation, via new *language games* in emergent dialogue—shared practices of speaking through which experience becomes newly describable, enlivened, and subjectively significant.[1]

Each chapter examines a different way language can become stuck in analytic dialogue. Conversation may fall into repetitive grooves, collapse into silence, or narrow into binary demands for certainty. Patients may search for

DOI: 10.4324/9781003598534-1

decisive insights or the "right words" that promise relief. By exploring these impasses, the chapters show how analytic work can loosen rigid language games and open space for new practices—ways of finding meaning together.

For Wittgenstein, words do not derive their meaning from what they claim to represent. Indeed, he argued that language does not directly represent inner states at all; "having a thought" is not literal reportage. Language gains its meaning from the roles our words play in shared activities or forms of life. It is not a "neutral" medium, like radio airwaves through which inner states are "transmitted"; rather, it is the means of *lived activity* through which experience becomes intelligible. Consider, for instance, teen or online slang, memes, rap lyrics, 12-step slogans, or quotations from contemporary analysts, which can sound nonsensical to those unfamiliar with the practices in which they are said.

Psychoanalysis, understood in this light, is not simply a method for revealing hidden truths, but a *setting* in which analyst and patient develop newly reflective ways of speaking about experience: new *grammars* of understanding, against the arising backdrop of the dyad itself.

Grammar is Wittgenstein's term for the background context or "genre" of speech, be it academic, cultural, familial, romantic, or analytic. Tennis culture is different from the culture of bridge, track and field, or professional poker. Even "sharing a thought" is a move within a language game; inner life and its subjective import are clarified through practices of expression easily taken for granted.

Patients often begin treatment with language games shaped in constrained environments, where emotional life was dismissed or disavowed, the language of emotionality flat or deadened. In these worlds, subjective experience becomes difficult, dangerous, or even pointless to articulate. There is no music here, only a hypnotic hum, like the quiet buzz of a refrigerator.

The patient may have grown up sensing their own painful blockages of speech, without an ability to name it. What later analytic theory has described as the unformulated (Stern, 2003) or unvalidated unconscious (Stolorow & Atwood, 1992) can be understood, in Wittgensteinian terms, as regions of experience lacking a workable grammar: a deeply unfamiliar game.

Analysis thus becomes less a process of excavation than one of negotiation, a verbalized sifting through: a new kind of practice, including for analysts learning to hear their patients. Through the rhythms of the dialogic, analysts help patients hear themselves and others from subtly different positions, loosening the grip of either/or framings. "Love," for instance, might no longer appear only as compliance. Patients slowly recognize a long-masked perspective staring them in the face: *their own.*

Expression becomes enlivened over time, and not *only* frightening. In speaking differently, patients begin to notice *family resemblances* (Wittgenstein, 2009) among uses of words, rather than searching for a single defining essence. Perhaps "care" from others does not *automatically* mean obligation, or "obligation" itself becomes negotiable. In this way analysts help patients broaden or shift the wrappings of the well-worn verbal straitjackets inherited early.

Aspects of subjectivity, once mute, begin to speak between the cracks of what had seemed monolithic.

Wittgenstein was intrigued by psychoanalytic ideas, admiring Freud's creatively astute interpretations of mental life; Freud was also a gifted writer and sensitive to the power of language, stating that "words were originally magic and to this day words have retained much of their ancient magical power" (1963, p. 17).

Yet Wittgenstein resisted Freud's archaeological model and its notions of what happens "within" the unconscious: the repressed meanings "buried" beneath thought. (Wittgenstein remained skeptical of speaking about *literal* mental processes.) The "unconscious" for Wittgenstein becomes another language game, a grammar more aesthetic than scientific.

Such matters were not trivial for Wittgenstein. They engaged him obsessively—a lifetime's quest, with an urgency inseparable from his life experience, shaped in part by his voluntary service at the front lines during the First World War.

This eccentric thinker endlessly puzzled over *what* is reliably conveyed in our everyday language games, how our shared practices make sense, and the constitutive grammar of our worlds. Such intensity parallels many analysts' commitment to understanding patients whose most painful struggles remain difficult or frightening to speak of, clouded by indistinct yet influential backgrounds.

Analysts, too, hope to be heard and understood—*acknowledged* may be the better term—by colleagues and patients alike: an underlying desire for efficacy (and recognition of same) often spoken of only obliquely among us. Our theories function like families in some respect, as the late Donna Orange (2014) reminds us. "My convictions do form a system, a structure," Wittgenstein writes (1969, § 102); patients' systems may hold beliefs apparently antithetical to those we have adopted and perhaps come to cherish, especially as such systems are "not so much the point of departure as the element in which arguments have their life" (1969, § 105).

Analysis, in other words, does not so much "uncover" meaning as *create the conditions under which meaning takes shape in speech.* The dialogic becomes a midwife to selfhood.

For families like Wittgenstein's, any such midwife is banished to the basement. Three of his brothers killed themselves, two of these deaths attributed to the domineering force of their father, Karl, an industrial magnate and one of the wealthiest men in Europe. Karl insisted on the peremptory belief that technical solutions existed for all of life's problems, and that his sons had a duty to succeed within the machinery of industrial capitalism (McGuiness, 1988). They instead longed for artistic lives he dismissed as impractical, even useless.

After these losses, Karl softened, a bit (McGuiness, 1988). Ludwig, the youngest of nine children, was a shy and awkward child, and did not speak until the age of four—significant, given that Wittgenstein would go on to claim that "the limits of my language are the limits of my world" (2013, § 5.6).

Meanwhile he was a mediocre student, who stammered and kept to himself. His mother Leopoldine cultivated an extraordinary cultural life within the home, hosting musicians such as Mahler and Brahms for recitals and private lessons.

Wittgenstein in adulthood vehemently rejected such pomp and splendor, pursuing life with monk-like austerity, including a ruthless honesty often unsolicited. He suffered no fools, including himself, despairing that philosophy demanded an uncompromising seriousness he feared he lacked. This led him to avoid almost any comfort made possible by the immense fortune he inherited and gave away, *in toto*, between World Wars (Monk, 1990). (Rilke was among the beneficiaries.)

He also rebuffed the frilled "perks" of academic society, sometimes turning his back to the audience who proffered the speaking invitation he (always reluctantly) accepted. He acted characteristically aloof toward a lover, while the latter was alive, later wailing like a banshee at the young man's funeral (a casualty of war), startling attendees (Monk, 1990).

Merciless toward muddled thinking—his own included—he later attempted awkward "apology tours" to atone for downplaying his Jewish ancestry in younger days. Such apologies co-existed with rageful outbursts. (I suspect Wittgenstein was on the autistic spectrum.)

What remained constant throughout these contradictions was the ferocity of his philosophical commitment, his one true partner. He tended to alienate everyone else.

Before the First World War, Wittgenstein studied at Cambridge under Bertrand Russell, who quickly recognized the brilliance of the intense young Austrian and affectionately referred to him as "my German" (Monk, 1990). Russell's encouragement helped stabilize Wittgenstein during a period when he was contemplating suicide.

The relationship later strained. Wittgenstein insisted that Russell misunderstood the *Tractatus Logico-Philosophicus* (2013), the first and only book published in Wittgenstein's lifetime. The book's introduction, provided by Russell himself, secured its publication; Wittgenstein later disparaged Russell's text. At his doctoral examination—where Russell served on the committee—Wittgenstein reportedly concluded the proceedings by remarking to said committee, "Don't worry, I know you'll never understand it" (MacFarlane, 2011).

The reader may be wondering what Wittgenstein's passionate focus on language has to do with analysis or analytic psychotherapy.[2]

Quite a bit, it turns out.

It continues to surprise me that so little of our analytic literature focuses on language and its fallible dynamics, given the linguistic turn in philosophy over the last century. Philosophers across the twentieth century, from Wittgenstein and Austin to Derrida and Foucault, have explored how meaning emerges *within* rather than outside linguistic practices.

Some psychoanalytic interest in this seismic turn include (among others) Stolorow, Atwood, Orange, Bollas, Heaton, LaPlanche, Bion, Maria Balaska (a former psychologist and now philosopher), Shawver—and of course Jacques Lacan, who famously proclaimed that "the unconscious is structured like a language," and that "the very foundation of interhuman discourse is misunderstanding" (both in Fink, 2014, p. 23). Lacan also describes subjectivity as positioned *within* practices of speech (the *symbolic realm,* he called it), rather than being uncovered or brought to light. We are always already positioned in networks of language systems, *born* into them, the oceans in which we swim.

Wilfrid Bion, who like Wittgenstein served in the First World War[3] as a tank commander, writes sensitively of the limitations of language in conveying the depths and contours of experience (including dreams). He cautions analysts against adopting shibboleths for the sake of the certainty we may seek, with a koan-like encouragement to practice without memory or desire (Grotstein, 2018).

Bion also shares Wittgenstein's skepticism that language alone conveys the nuance needed for understanding, especially when cloaked in rationality and habit (and our analytic assumptions): "In psychoanalysis, we have to manufacture our means of communicating *while we are communicating"* (1975, p. 31, italics mine).

The classical tradition, the founders of psychoanalysis, communicate to us in *literary* form; Freud was greatly aided by his formidable writing skills. The rest continue to speak via the papers, books, and lectures of our forebears, to say nothing of the voluminous commentary following in their wake.

Yet very little in our literature, relatively speaking, focuses on the functions of language itself, the underlying dynamics informing the analytic project. Ironic, given the text-centricity of said enterprise, starting with Freud's *talking cure;* such talking, Balaska (2019) points out, is "addressed to another being, as an attempt to…understand and be understood…subject to the logical/normative conditions of language" (p. 215).

Each familial, sociocultural, and dyadic context carries its own sense of what counts as "normative"—parallel or competing backgrounds—complicating matters from the start (no one said it would be easy). Additionally, Wittgenstein comments enquiries must start somewhere, resting on what he calls hinge agreements (1969), or propositional "givens", that "all enquiry on our part is set so as to exempt certain propositions from doubt … They lie apart from the route travelled by enquiry" (1969, § 88). For instance, the assumption that analysis is a worthy endeavor, a valuation more shown or *demonstrated* than said or explained.

Words are powerful, seductive, risking what Wittgenstein called "the bewitchment of our intelligence by means of language" (2009, § 109). Theory can stiffen into slogans or quiet shibboleths, further annexing the tender challenge of tolerating uncertainty.

Wittgenstein (2009) observes how our language games traverse familiarity with repetition, settling into intuition after a time—from rough to well-trodden ground. Analytic traction often slips on thin ice. *How did we get here?* Wittgenstein likened philosophy to drawing a map, to help us find our way "out of the flybottle" (2009, § 309). Such maps require constant revision, since even ordinary language games—never mind psychoanalysis—are surprisingly complicated. Analysts overlook the complexity of our clinical cartography, in helping patients sketch a map of their own minds, including long-unnoticed, cordoned-off neighborhoods. Or, with more intellectually defended patients, they can name the neighborhoods by heart, even if they have never visited them (theory can work this way, too).

All of this underlines a view of language as a *practice*: fluid and co-constructed. Wittgenstein stubbornly resisted conceptual solidity, metaphysics, or scientism, their use as bulwarks against uncertainty. Ethical orientations, too, he suggests in his *Lecture on Ethics* (1993), are largely *lived* rather than stated, shown rather than said. He was skeptical that ethical values could be "proved" in language alone.

Wittgenstein's seminal *Philosophical Investigations* (2009) is, for the most part, a series of questions with occasional answers, metaphors, and analogies designed to provoke our reflective wheels, a playful yet serious game with different voices and interlocutors—a living demonstration of the miracle that is language (rather than using language to define the miraculous (Wittgenstein, 1993)).

This might of course prove rather flimsy for a patient hoping in her agony that the analyst will "know" precisely what to do, what actions to prescribe to ward off suffering. (Take two affirmations and call me in the morning.) As one patient, struggling with imploding romances and disordered eating, asked after a week into analysis, "Now that you know all my traumas, how do I move on?" I often find myself wondering what my expertise consists of, in speakable terms, contingent of course on who is listening.

How to convey the *significance* (to who?) of *what* is so often shameful or aversive to speak of; a patient's long-dormant selfhood may have value *we alone* may recognize for the longest time. We cannot get any patient to "see" anything, least of all via explanation—only to attempt to suggest or evoke novel notions, widened perspectives. As Gadamer puts it, "Understanding or its failure is like an event *that happens to us*" (2013, p. 401, italics mine).

In a later work on psychology, Wittgenstein discusses the classic duck-rabbit optical illusion, where we notice one and then the other, without knowing why or how this shift occurs. He calls this shift the "lighting up of an aspect" (in Lemberger, 2017, p. 197); it is impossible to explain *precisely* what "leads to" such shifts, analogous to our work with patients archaically coerced into seeing only the rabbit while ignoring the duck, the latter loudly obvious to us.

Rigid, addictive, or accommodative self-organizations can remain hostile to the fluidity of our hermeneutic project (e.g., *I alone am the problem,* an attitude that analysts may find themselves slipping into). Here I mean those alcoholic, narcissistic, or otherwise subjugating systems that disallow the patients to be who they are or hope to be (Shaw, 2014), the expansion of personalized expression. Such expressiveness is taboo, leading to the entrenched self-descriptions of one's inadequacy or selfishness, problematic descriptions postponing solutions. Affect becomes thing-like, to be discarded or "rewired" like a machine. *Got any tools for existential angst, Doc?*

Hard to forget the patient who blandly asked for tools facilitating "sexy thoughts" about the wife who criticized him nonstop—even in bed, where he struggled to attain an erection. He talked of this blandly, like the weather—his languaging, too, drained of blood. He refused the idea that such bodily withdrawal might serve a purpose.

In such scenarios, psychic conflict arises when "one is not aware that the deep problems one sets out to tackle are side effects of the language used to think of them" (Cimatti, 2015, p. 242). The problem preserved self-blame and (perhaps) the adhesive dynamics of the marriage itself. "Sexy thoughts" were treated like ingredients in a recipe the patient desired but could not name, "failure" the only recognizable item (flavorless but reliable). He soon fell off the radar completely.

Wittgenstein viewed philosophy as a therapy for lingual confusion, as, for instance, seeking the "core explanation" for depression, addiction, a dream, or wounded longing, cited from a manual we surely have stashed under our chairs—versus a *found way* of describing it. In our current era, everything (or nothing) invites the diagnostic. Wittgenstein states that confusing grammar and reified concepts (e.g., that analysis can "cure") are like "an illness" (2009, § 255) or "mental cramps" (1958, p. 59), these "sicknesses of … understanding" (1967, §382).

Terms like "treatment" or "understanding" hold different values to different participants; all patients speak a dialect our ears strain to learn. There is often required of me, as illustrated in vignettes throughout this volume, a painful realignment (Brandchaft, 1993) of assumptions I have made, as "work on philosophy is really more work on oneself … on how one sees things" (Wittgenstein, 1998, p. 24). There is no easier, softer way.[4]

Consider a speech more literal than metaphoric: two perspectives separated by a common language. How to translate *any* metaphor as a bridge between body and mind, fundamental to discerning meanings (Lakoff & Johnson, 1980), made real in clinical practice? Even *subjectivity* represents a framing of unrecognized import to those trapped within the "tyranny of fixed horizons and frozen meaning" (Orange, 2002, p. 693).

Often such frozenness, lingual narcotization, rigidly grips addictive systems (as in my own upbringing). The fierce denial of a caregiver vaporizes the child's lived reality; here naming the addiction is of greater offense than the abuse itself, as if the child's words held destructive power, for which they are solely responsible (such words spoken, after all, by them alone).

These chokeholds against emotionality remain influential well into treatment. Any acknowledgment of influence ("my folks did what they could, I'm over it now") is iced over with unnamable entrapment.

What participants tend to seek, in my view, are language games bearing distinctive *family resemblances* to each other, where "naming a feeling" becomes narrativized, idiomatically signified rather than distantly "factual." Analysis offers the possible co-creation of a *blended family,* for all the promise and peril this implies.

Balaska's *Wittgenstein and Lacan at the Limit* (2019), her useful study of language and our creative use of it, parallels the philosophical and psychoanalytic, in stating that "it is *in the recognition of servitude that the possibility for freedom becomes available* …." (Balaska, 2019, p. 155, italics mine).

It is the need for clinical creativity with words, in pushing past the confining limits of constraint that propelled the writing of this book. The first step is speaking to and around the edges that Balaska outlines.

What makes this difficult is our losing sight of our tranquilizing familiarity with language, where "we use it but we are not aware of using it. It seems as if there was no language between us and the world" (Cimatti, 2015, p. 241). We might even be lulled into perceiving clinical essences as sensed or heard; it appears in the end simply, fallibly human to hold that "one is tracing the outline of the thing's nature over and over again, when one is merely *tracing round the frame through which we look at it*" (Wittgenstein, 2009, § 114, italics mine).

We cannot see the frame through which experience undergoes aspect-shifts; in a sense we *are* the frame. Even recognizing pain is an embedded practice of call and response as "you learned the concept 'pain' when you learned language" (2009, § 384). A child learns via response that "ow!" carries *lived* value, a word worth hearing. (Cavell states that "your suffering makes a claim upon me" (2002, p. 243), recognition a shared form of life.)

In democratizing the dialogic via the relational turn, contemporizing theorists discerned new ways of describing unconscious processes. Stephen Mitchell (2000) and Donnell Stern (2009, 2003) establish a framework of the *relational unconscious* and *unformulated* experience, respectively—established in clinically lived dialogue. Prior to such dialogue, such processes remain unformulated, incipiently enlivened into the currents of analytic discourse.

This in parallel (a family resemblance) to Stolorow and Atwood's (1992) *unvalidated unconscious,* archaic experiences whose traumatic impact (or existence) went acknowledged. These authors compare such invalidation to scraps of building materials in an abandoned basement. (Many have felt just like this.)

It is worth pausing for a moment over the grammar of *the* unformulated or unvalidated. What exactly is the article indicating here? Wittgenstein reminds us that an inner process "stands in need of outward criteria" (2009, § 580), and elsewhere remarks that such private sensations are "not a something, but not a nothing either!" (§ 304). The definite article, *the*, functions less as a description than as a pointer—an arrow on the map of experience indicating something not yet sketched in. In this sense the unformulated is not a hidden object awaiting discovery but a *possibility for articulation*, calling upon patients' participation, inscriptions in their own hand.

The same applies to recognizing the *what* and *how* of dissociative processes. *What* is being dissociated, appearing absently present? Again we are visualizing steam, as both participants periodically face a "break with the idea that language always functions in one way, always serves the same purpose" (Wittgenstein, 2009, § 304). Perhaps—patients often suggest—such affective "steam" is best left alone, not worth hearing, a stillbirth. Such disorientation can, once we reconstitute, help us recognize a patient's isolating silence; we become what many of my patients describe (and as we may have once experienced), the child watching other kids play from the sidelines—the unsayable loneliness of peremptory observing. Thus it becomes difficult to induce patients to *get in the game.*

We initiate patients into our analytic perspectives, induct them into our private practices, more than we acknowledge; perhaps doing so threatens the notion of semi-neutrality (an idea of surprising potency), of parking our concerns on the "backburner"—except of course those concerns of investiture leading us to the analyst's chair.

Wittgenstein questions these temptations, to previsualize the boil in the pot with a certainty bordering on the predictive, via a deceptively simple example:

> If water boils in a pot, steam comes out of the pot and also pictured steam comes out of the pictured pot. But what if one insisted on saying that there must also be something boiling in the picture of the pot?
>
> (2009, § 297)

Wittgenstein's example captures the seduction of "seeing" prereflective meaning as akin to secluded objects awaiting a flashlight. It also reveals something subtler: what appears as hidden may instead await *articulation*, via the language games generating aspect-shifts of perspective.

So much analytic theory (starting with Freud) leads us to visualize that boil, awaiting a cursory lifting of the lid. *Where is the grief, the rage, the pain...* we may wonder, knowing it is "there" somewhere. Is it? More difficult to sit with the strange nothing-but-still-something quality of stirrings elusive to words.

The vagueness of prearticulated affect leads some patients to ask *how* we know (or can prove) that any such steam is "really" there. Who is to say, some remark, that dreams "mean" anything at all, or that so-called unconscious influences "exist," are not antiquated, fanciful, or quaint? Better to trust the inky scratches of a brain-scan.

I often take these things as self-evident: *of course dreams mean something!* Such questions sound absurd, even insulting. But this has led over time—given the sincerity of patients' confusions or skepticism toward the intangible (and our cultural leaning on the tangible)—to wondering *how* I have come to believe in the significance of dreams and unconscious processes, their usefulness to us, and how subsequently to talk about them to the uninitiated. (Most new patients still equate analysis with a pipe, divan, and beard.)

Our craving for general explanations can seduce us into believing that once a mechanism is identified, its meaning speaks for itself. In contemporary psychology this temptation is often via the neuroscientific. We are repeatedly in mainstream journalism invited to "trust the science" of human existence in such a way (fascinating as much of it is). The danger lies in hearing these statements as guarantees, as if neural activity "shows" the significance of a dream, of human subjectivity.

But then, how much can we (or ought we) defend our forms of analytic life? At some point explanations come to an end, Wittgenstein reminds us; our shovel hits rock, and we are inclined to say, "this is simply what I do" (2009, § 217). Patients tend to want what we offer—*buy in,* as it were—or not.

That forms of analytic *practice* is all we do have is, at times, tough to swallow. Alternative perspectives even within our field, spoken with a certainty equal to mine (again forgotten in the flow of life), can tremor the very ground. Our acknowledging change is not the same as accepting its implications, as new generations and perspectives remind us that "at the core of all well-founded belief lies belief that is unfounded" (1969, § 153). (It is, however, practiced in language games and grammar we become reliant upon.)

This is the great tension of language, the impulse to understand versus tolerating twilight, sitting with (or even in) the possibility of incomprehension. We might even say meaning *finds us,* in a Gadamerian sense, amidst our investigations, swimming upstream, against the currents of a compulsion to *know*—as if, at edgier moments, the correct words will open the portal stubbornly locked. (Though sometimes it is helpful to know just what to say.)

It gnaws deeply at us, with patients who find enigmatic their own compulsive self-destruction, our longing for a placeholder against self-erasure, while lacking any explanation of heft; especially unnerving this is, to those who have lost patients (as I have) to suicide, overdose, or other dark chaos. If we cannot yet know, let us at least acknowledge the danger.

Cavell captures this tension, the urgency of Wittgenstein's project:

> That on the whole we do [understand each other] is a matter of our sharing routes of interest and feeling, modes of response, senses of humor and of significance and of fulfillment, of what is outrageous…what a rebuke,

> what forgiveness...all the whirl of organism Wittgenstein calls "forms of life." Human speech and activity, sanity and community, rest upon nothing more, but nothing less, than this. It is a vision as simple as it is difficult, and as difficult as it is (and because it is) terrifying.
>
> (2002, p. 48)

What is terrifying is what often drives enactments; in certain conflicts our existence seems threatened; looming is the threatened permanence of severed connection. This relates to a notion of Lacan's, who describes naming an other is akin to "the murder of the thing" (2001/1977, p. 114), a presence of absence taken up by language, which absence allows it to function. Starting with *mama* or *dada,* our words embed in the very separation that enables them. This is the melancholic nature of the symbolically spoken, borne by division, engendered by an absence and longing, perhaps, for a return to the literally embodied, a time where alphabetic symbols were unnecessary. (Sexual activity may later—briefly, persuasively—fill this gap.)

Our bodies of language, in other words, gradually replace the corporeal in our symbolic development. Inherent in speech is the desire for (re)unification, a compulsion to be met in word and deed—thwarted for some via language games malignly enforced from early days. Environments hard of hearing promote the safety of dissociative existence. Such a systemically peremptory, inverted discourse (prioritizing the other) (Lacan, 2001) erases the potential for a lyrical versus literal symbolizing, in one's own dialect, sometimes with near-finality. Even the grief of separation or loss collapses inward, an unbearable solitude also unspoken.

Analysts may be tempted to leap past such frightful chasms, that yawning vastness, a blank page whose emptiness might be permanent, keening for the inscription of a narrative of the patient's own. *Will history repeat?*

Wittgenstein faced his own chasm, that of his demise (speaking of terrifying), with typical austerity. For his 62nd birthday he received a gift from a friend who wished him many happy returns. "There will be no returns!" he declared, dead a few days later. "Tell them I've had a wonderful life," he said, before slipping into the ether, claimed in finality by prostate cancer (both quotes in Monk, 1990, p. 579).

He wrote as he lived, wrestling with ways language is always pursuing but never quite catching up to the complexities of co-existence. Dialogue with patients, along with the language of our theory worlds, follows on the mercurial heels of lived experience; the proverbial dog after the car.

Eventually, though, the dog bites, or tries to. Our craving for generality (Wittgenstein, 1958) gives way to the ambiguity of the specific. We learn to speak in rhythm, within the tenor of our combined language games, whose purpose sometimes reveals itself in contrasts, occasionally jarring: those gaps of difference that allow us to locate resemblances hiding in plain sight.

Notes

1 Stolorow and Atwood (1992) similarly criticize the tendency in some psychoanalytic traditions to treat the self as a thing-like structure, rather than as a phenomenological term denoting selfhood-in-context.
2 I will use the two interchangeably throughout for the sake of concision, recognizing obvious differences too complicated to explicate here.
3 Bion later remarked that he died in 1918 on a battlefield in France, in a violently chaotic tank battle, where friends and fellow soldiers were blown to bits before his eyes (Grotstein, 2018).
4 This is a slogan often heard in recovery meetings.

References

Balaska, M. (2019). *Wittgenstein and Lacan at the limit: Meaning and astonishment.* Palgrave Macmillan.

Bion, W.R. (1975). *Bion's Brazilian lectures.* Imago Editoria.

Brandchaft, B. (1993). To free the spirit from its cell. *Progress in Self Psychology*, (9):209–230.

Cavell, S. (2002). *Must we mean what we say?* Cambridge University Press. Originally published 1969.

Cimatti, F. (2015). Philosophy and psychoanalysis: Wittgenstein, on 'language-games' and ethics. In A. Capone & J.L. Mey (Eds.), *Interdisciplinary studies in pragmatics, culture and society* (*perspectives in pragmatics, philosophy & psychology*) (Vol. 4, pp. 233–250.). Springer.

Fink, B. (2014). Against understanding: Cases and commentary in a Lacanian key. Routledge.

Freud, S. (1963). *Introductory lectures on psychoanalysis* (J. Strachey, Ed. & Trans.) W.W. Norton. Originally published 1916.

Gadamer, H. (2013). *Truth and method* (J. Weinsheimer & D.G. Marshall, Trans.) Bloomsbury Academic. Originally published 1975.

Grotstein, J. (2018). *A beam of intense darkness: Wilfred Bion's legacy to psychoanalysis.* Routledge. Originally published 2007.

Lacan, J. (2001). *Ecrits: A selection* (A. Sheridan, Trans.) Routledge Classics. Originally published 1977.

Lakoff, G., & Johnson, M. (1980). Metaphors We Live By. Chicago: University of Chicago Press.

Lemberger, D. (2017). Wittgenstein's 'lighting up of an aspect' and the possibility of change in psychoanalytic therapy. *British Journal of Psychotherapy*, 33(2):192–210.

MacFarlane, L. (2011). *Ludwig Wittgenstein: 1889–1951. Philosophy now* [blog article]. Retrieved from https://philosophynow.org/issues/87/Ludwig_Wittgenstein_1889-1951

Mitchell, S. (2000). *Relationality.* Routledge.

McGuiness, B. (1988). *Wittgenstein: A life (Young Ludwig: 1889–1921).* University of California Press.

Monk, R. (1990). *Ludwig Wittgenstein: The duty of genius.* Penguin.

Orange, D.M. (2002). There is no outside: Empathy and authenticity in psychoanalytic process. *Psychoanalytic Psychology*, 19(4):686–700.

Orange, D.M. (2014). And we shall be changed: To hold theory lightly is to surrender assumptions: Discussion of clinical narrative by Steven Stern. *International Journal of Psychoanalytic Self Psychology*, 9(3):193–199.

Shaw, D. (2014). Traumatic Narcissism: Relational systems of subjugation. Routledge.

Stern, D.B. (2003). *Unformulated experience: From dissociation to imagination in psychoanalysis*. Analytic Press (Relational Perspectives).

Stern, D.B. (2009). *Partners in thought: Working with unformulated experience, dissociation, and enactment*. Routledge.

Stolorow, R.D., & Atwood, G.E. (1992). *Contexts of being: The intersubjective foundations of everyday life*. Analytic Press (Relational Perspectives).

Wittgenstein, L. (1958). *The blue and brown books: Preliminary studies for the 'philosophical investigations.'* Blackwell Publishing.

Wittgenstein, L. (1967). *Zettel* (G. E. M. Anscombe, Trans.; G. E. M. Anscombe & G. H. von Wright, Eds.). University of California Press.

Wittgenstein, L. (1969). *On certainty* (D. Paul, & G.E.M. Anscombe, Trans.) (G.E.M. Anscombe, & G.H. Von Wright, Eds.) Basil Blackwell.

Wittgenstein, L. (1993). A lecture on ethics. In J. Klagge & A. Nordmann (Eds.), *Philosophical occasions 1912–1951* (pp. 37–44). Hackett Publishing Company.

Wittgenstein, L. (1998). *Culture & value* (P. Winch, Trans.) (G.H. Von Wright, & H. Nyman, Eds.) Blackwell Publishers Ltd. Originally published 1977.

Wittgenstein, L. (2009). *Philosophical investigations* (4th ed.) (G.E.M. Anscombe, P.M.S. Hacker, & J. Schulte, Trans.) (P.M.S. Hacker, & J. Schulte, Eds.) Blackwell Publishing Ltd. Originally published 1953.

Wittgenstein, L. (2013). *Tractatus logico-philosophicus* (C.K. Ogden, & F.P. Ramsey, Trans.). e-artnow (Kindle edition). Originally published 1922.

2 Dissociation and Language Games in Psychoanalysis

Struck Dumb

Captive Phrases

If language is indeed at "the heart of human dwelling" (Hatab, 2017, p. 118), how to address the void of a shattered heart, in ways that cannot be co-acknowledged, spoken of, or even recognized as significant in dyadic process? How to address a presence characterized by a perseverant absence?

In this chapter, I address such absences in the context of addiction, a specialty of mine, where compulsive avoidance of troublesome affect becomes an entrenched way of life, such aversion eventually becoming unseen and de-registered even in sobriety.

I remember my analyst asking a question, early in treatment, that I was ashamed I couldn't answer, in regard to negotiating some of the challenges of early marriage. I was struck dumb, surprised that couples could talk about such things. It was hard to imagine what words to use—honest but not demanding, candid but not critical, flexible yet … *Ugh.* Mostly I could not pin down *why such speech eluded me.*

I could not yet discern, in other words, at that stage of my own recovery, how difficult it was to inhabit my own agency, smothered in younger days by demands for accommodation, including the ability to recognize such smothering. It also took time to see what "agency" even meant, subjectively.

Case Study: Keep Coming Back

As analyst John Heaton notes, "It is the specific features of a person's language that correspond to its untranslatable expressions" (Heaton, 2013, p. 122).

Jonathan had been sober in AA for ten or so years, finding sober success in all areas except dating. His sponsor suggested therapy,

DOI: 10.4324/9781003598534-2

given that he was nearly middle-aged and had yet to find lasting romance. His relationships tended to be erotically charged but brief.

His latest conflagration involved another volatile affair that recently imploded, initiated by a woman who pursued him. The pursuit thrilled him until he discovered she was frequently "prickly." When he got up the gumption to protest, she accused him of neediness. She then "ghosted" him, ignoring his "needy" (he said) messages, before she sent him a furious breakup text.

He anguished over whether to apologize, missing the sex but not the drama. When I asked what he missed about sex, he grinned and said, "Dude, c'mon." (A cigar was just a cigar.)

Jonathan knew about my recovery background, hopeful I could help. He was well-respected in his meetings, sponsoring several young men who admired him. But he carried an odd detachment; life seemed to just … happen, all around him.

Jonathan believed his romantic "picker" was broken, "thanks to my pecker." He described himself as "full of self-will, codependence and character defects." This to me was generic recovery language, though he seemed to believe this said it all.

I sensed this patient hated himself, but that any source of self-loathing was also conceptualized: "Self-loathing is a form of self-will," he said, before repeating his favorite mantra: "The problem is in the mirror." But whose gaze looked back?

Jonathan was bright and dedicated, and sobriety is not always easy. He had just opened a successful sober living house for young men, who were as lost as he had been in more youthful days.

He found alcohol in his teens, finally escaping a surrogate spousehood to a volatile, alcoholic father. Here, the "rules" of accommodation were written in stone, even as Wittgenstein (2009) describes even the rules of our games as context-dependent. But if Jonathan said the wrong thing, was a bit too honest or unfiltered, his dad exploded with rage and criticism. This established Jonathan's spontaneity as dangerous, no matter the context, dovetailing later with his reliance on recovery sayings.

The model scene had young Jonathan mute on the floor, drawing or reading comics, while his father drank on the couch—the TV chattering between them.

But soon I felt hostage to such thickened silence, as notions of empathy and connectivity seemed not to register with a man I felt to be very lonely, de-centered in an ability to speak of or dwell in his isolation. Why bother, if he knew it would change nothing? Meantime he chalked up his romantic indecision over Shannon to "addiction to excitement" and "not trusting God," as if AA expects perfection rather than progress (yet "humility is not humiliation" is also a slogan).

Often there were awkward clinical silences, me searching for ways to engage. Jon said he enjoyed our meetings, though he did most of the talking, which I at times found hard to follow given its subjective de-centering. In a way, any subjectivity was problematic.

Still, I was reluctant to rain on his parade and remembered a therapist from early sobriety who mocked "the scriptures of AA," which I found arrogant and discouraging. So I kept my frustrations to myself, overcorrecting perhaps, inadvertently hiding from Jonathan, which also kept him hidden from view.

Jonathan could not stop ruminating in binary fashion on whether to try again with Shannon, recalling her praising his attractiveness and their passionate lovemaking, leading to anguished self-doubt due to his "codependence" and certain "love addiction," connected to the "highs" of feeling desired.

I responded that there were underlying reasons for "codependence," such as yearnings due to abandonment; he sincerely responded that yes, abandonment leads to codependence, which "doesn't mean you can just indulge." The end.

Sometimes he sounded angry at Shannon, emotion hurried into the wings or flagged for "indulgence." The problem is in the mirror. Anger is described as dangerous in AA, linked with relapse and death. I would say to this basically, "Ok fair enough, but you still sound angry … perhaps hurt," in other words, human. "So what do we do about it," he would immediately respond. I said here that we were already "doing" quite a bit. This seemed not to satisfy him.

I was not sure what he hoped to receive from me, as he again repeated he enjoyed our meetings. Was this accommodation? Our work felt nowhere near "analytic."

Clearly, accommodation was at work here for both of us. Jones (2009) describes demands for conformity in *some* corners of the program, a rigidity that devalues affectivity in favor of rule-following (possibly quite helpful for some at the beginning).

AA's ideas of addiction, Jones points out, evolved from a classical one-person psychology, framing addiction as a failure of personal accountability. (The problem is in the mirror.)

Some accommodation is probably necessary or even vital in the early days, but rigidity of any stripe can lead to dogmatism. Discovering intersubjective systems, its description of traumatic contexts, was emancipating, at a time when my own sponsor was dismissive of psychotherapy. I reluctantly dropped him.

Jonathan had a different relationship to these familiar words and terms that, as I saw, kept him both sober and distant from his affective world and the value of its expression. "Come on in," I wanted to say, "the water's warm!" But he appeared compelled to stay landlocked.

I gamely tried translating notions of the affectivity of trauma and eroticized desire into language related to recovery, sex as a "remedy" for toxic hurt and shame.

"That's the codependence!" he exclaimed. I heard a book slamming shut.

I once wondered aloud, with deliberate gentleness, if he remembered much about the mother who left when he was two.

He shrugged. "She did the best she could. She needed Al-anon. It's sad."

"Yes," I said. "Sad."

I wondered if he ever felt angry at his father. He laughed. "My dad never got the gift! Gotta have compassion for the alcoholic who still suffers." But what about little Jonathan? "I'm sober," he said, "and lucky. I turned out fine."

Yet he seemed frustrated at his inability to think or talk himself out of desiring Shannon, another Rubik's cube. He often asked what to "do" about this. I responded we were doing it now. He said, "And how does that help?" The question felt vaguely like a jab. I responded that we had to pause, parse what his emotions were "saying." He said we had already answered that; they said he was codependent.

How does one "explain" a relational perspective, the significance of one's own emotionality? Jonathan was certainly making an effort, once remarking, "I'm really digging in here." Still, I felt disavowed, wondering how my own contribution led us astray. The problem is in the mirror.

Then Shannon reappeared out of the blue, and his world went wobbly. "She's hinting she wants a reunion," he said. He said if sex was in the cards he was "definitely going for it," as if issuing a warning. Yet he hesitated.

He came close to fragmenting as sessions wore on, riven with conflict, insisting that sex was "intoxicating" yet "stupid" (or dangerous), though the craving persisted. He continued to shun aspects of his own subjectivity, reminding me that for an alcoholic everything was potentially addictive. I felt more and more boxed in.

How could I "get analytic" and sustain inquiry long enough to reach the vulnerability beneath? (As if there were such a "beneath.")

He sheepishly admitted that Shannon had an "amazing ass." I said, "Nothing wrong with that … but aren't there plenty of asses in the sea? Why not someone less critical?" "Because she approached me!" he said. So why not approach someone else? "Not until I fix this codependence!" "So why rush to see Shannon," I said. "Because she called me!" he said. I said, at wit's end, wondering where he was in all this, "Can you … not call back?"

"I'm getting very angry," he said, reddening, "you keep asking me over and over again and I've told you, again and again. It just keeps happening, my entire life, this whole fucking cycle, why is that not getting through?"

The match was lit, the room … *alive.*

I saw it then: *over and over*, night after night, him waiting for some crumb of there-ness with a father who numbed himself, barely noticing the boy on the floor … who surely, silently wondered, "What do I have to say to get some goddamn attention? I haven't spoken out of turn. I've been good!" In this way, his own foundational needs became toxic and later eroticized with women via a yearning ever shameful, an ouroboros of isolation.

Such desires were forbidden, even dreaded—buried beneath a contempt ever pointed at the unquestionable addictivity (or wrongness) of such desires. (So wrong yet so right, as the old saying goes.)

In Wittgenstein's terms, we were trapped in a particular language game in which feeling was indistinguishable from dangerous impulse; this contributed to Jonathan's shameful stuckness. In a survivalist preoccupation with the exterior—the outside and never the inside—the person's interior is embedded in the optics of objectivity, blurring any inner life of worth or speakability. (These are often intertwined.)

I told Jonathan he was right. He had answered me, and I had missed it, overlooked the fraught nature of his dilemma, and how was that for him? He murmured that he felt ignored. I imagined that was a sad, familiar feeling. He agreed … then said, "I have no idea what to do here." For the first time, I heard a kind of shameful terror over an "obvious" yes or no decision.

I reflected aloud that maybe sex versus no-sex was a red herring, a binary tripping us up. Perhaps the problem was not his wanting something that felt so good and turned out bad. The problem perhaps was his wanting … anything at all from someone else.

Because that something came from another, which had never been safe. So often his desire was paired with a dread of being viewed as inherently "gross." It was therefore scary to want something from Shannon, or even me. But it was likely impossible to turn off this deeply human want, including his passion for sex, a connection that was so thrillingly validating; in parallel, he hoped in therapy for an understanding of how to satisfy the divisions wrought by his erotic or *any* need. All of this left him in shameful confusion, as it really "shouldn't be that hard."

"Makes sense," he said, faintly smiling.

Then it dawned on me. How had I missed it? I said to him that sex must really be magical … a time he finally got to feel alive! In that sense, maybe, it was essential, motivating him toward life, feeling desired, a need safely held.

"That's it," he said. "I mean sex is amazing. But then …" "Yes. But then." I paused. "This is hard," I said.

"It is," he said, his face alighting into a smile, as if I had heard his very first words.

Concluding Thoughts

What we were somehow avoiding in our dialogue and its dark magnetism was the experience of nothing, or the experience of nothingness—the absence of a speakable inner life, a silent vastness gripping us both.

It can be daunting, overwhelming even, for patients to recognize just how much has been lost, as stirrings of tender but agonizing subjectivity come to life.

I sensed aftershocks of Jonathan's losses, amidst our lingual enactment, but could not speak to them in ways he might hear, because I did not yet know him, a gap that I recognized but needed time to address, forgetting I could not do so alone. For Jonathan this was an aridly conceptual process; we had yet to find our way, amidst gripping anxiety. Bewitchment filled the gap.

His own chasmic wounds were ameliorated ephemerally by sex, in its admixture of fantasized gratification and embodied pleasure. In the end, he could dismiss it; it's just sex. The roaring backgrounds of such yearnings were oceanic.

Our mutual angst was equally silent, let omniscient. I misread his use of AA slogans as absolutes, for me a paternal repetition of demands to accommodate rather than explore—bricks slammed to the table, erecting a wall. But for him they were a life preserver, in offering him a way to speak to his problem, even as they reinforced impossible ideals to self-correct.

Such formulations also protected him, unconsciously, from the terror of an unknown intersubjective process, in vulnerably wanting guidance. Here I felt blocked, as if again demanded to mind-read a well-protected other, lest I look incompetent, from "expert."

It turns out this was a dialogue of sorts for him, given his lifetime of isolation. I tend to define "dialogue" in the way I prefer, lively and engaged (the ex-New Yorker in me), not the molasses-like silences that often permeate. It is easy to miss the marginal whisperings amidst the drone of repetition.

Jonathan's use of recovery language unwittingly foreclosed my ability to imagine other ways to hear his statements (i.e., as bids to achieve ideals and subsequent approval). Missed by me was the underlying despair, from a man who felt compelled to live and speak "correctly," which he saw not as his perception of recovery but as "the truth," reinforced via the unsymbolized expectations of his sponsor and recovery peers.

Paternal repetition haunted the entire ambience.

Without his recognizing how profoundly his early caregiver system led to such expectations, his only conclusion was that his inadequacy in romantic relationships, another stinging belly-flop. Alongside this was the parallel terror of failing at therapy, suggested by his sponsor, a double nail in the coffin of self-esteem. This raised the stakes for both of us, leading me to lean in a bit too much, too soon.

This misdirected me from my representing another father for him, one who might save or scold or again shame rather than listen to him; the shadow of the archaic paternal object (Freud, 1917) falling across his strivings for guidance.

Yet this too was a detour; I could not provide anything substantive without understanding the very subjectivity he was compelled to de-couple. Additionally, some recovery slogans ask that participants "stop making this all about you," which out of context becomes another absolute. I *had* to make it about him, becoming restless and impatient as (I discovered belatedly) he had no idea what I was after, those more intimate language games or forms of life so familiar to me and taken for granted. For Jonathan, recovery had long been the only game in town.

Anxious to "get things moving," I then reached for explanations and descriptions of psychodynamic process, avoiding a look at our mutual angst. He said such explanations were helpful, perhaps because I sounded confident, but they only got us so far.

My repetitive fear of subjugation—toward recovery concepts, pried from my analytic home-world—exaggerated my perceptions of Jonathan's cloaked despair as another accommodation to the rules, as with my dad and former sponsor (who belittled therapy). Symbolization became a hostage to the concrete.

Only later could I describe our work to him as an "extended fourth step," a framing that eased us toward both/and rather than the either/or of recovery versus psychodynamics.

In fact, I initially suspected some unnamed transference afoot, underestimating the influence it was already wielding. Yet Saying to myself, "I may have paternal transference here" bestowed a superficial certainty, as if I knew what was what and could handle it accordingly, on my own, like the precociously self-reliant boy.

"Transference" too can be glossed, its depths overlooked. I resisted looking deeper because, well, I liked Jonathan, respected his recovery, feared the arising of annoyance or anger and becoming dismissive of him, as that former therapist had somewhat snidely done with me.

So I tried to meet the patient where he was, adapting a similar explanatory tone in "translating" the process of analytic therapy, the significance of emotion, the personal meaning of events, blah blah blah … as if I were speaking factually to "counter" objective statements, a chess game going nowhere.

Jonathan, for instance, would speculate that his trauma was linked to codependence. What did this mean? To him it meant what it said: a bypassing of the need to speak to his need, a move that spoke for itself. By this I mean he was failing yet again but did not know or had not been shown how to *get it right*, because "right" led to intolerable vulnerability. The answer was lived, not explained, itself difficult to explain.

I was not concerned about his anger at me (a spark of life!), so much as my own gnawing annoyance, lest I lose patience, become haughty or "unprofessional," *become* the deflating father. I also saw him as a kind of sibling I was loathe to disappoint, with residual shame over bullying my little brother in younger days, amidst family chaos: lurking elephants in an office smallish to begin with.

Jonathan, meanwhile, protected me from his "demands," as he had been taught to perceive them, like many neglected patients withholding their contemptuous need for help, lest they (re)enrage caregiver-figures.

Additionally, venting emotional distress in some pockets of recovery is frowned upon. "Fuck your feelings and don't drink," is the idea. Or, as one long-timer told me when I was new, "This ain't Alcoholics Analysis."

Taken out of context, such statements become bewitchments of recovery language, a topic beyond the scope of this chapter. It serves to remind us however of the danger of generalization, instead of interrogating our need for certainty and the context of use or need. What was true for me in the beginning did not remain so ten years later. Even now, we may need to "keep it simple," or dig in, depending on circumstance.

But again, generalizations are impossible to avoid entirely. We remind ourselves, for instance, to hold our theory lightly (Orange, 2014). But should we ever hold *this* lightly? How do we "know" theory, furthermore? Perhaps we recognize something in it, a resonance within our own subjectivity, drawing us into a perspective, as much an acknowledgment as a knowing (Wittgenstein, 1969), as with clinical observations and interpretations, a framing of what we see before us.

We get lost in the centrifuge of repetition, as with a new patient seeking description of our "expertise," in a language or perspective we hope to translate to a person new to us. We do know something, based on work with patients, but not this patient and their idiomatic point of view (Bollas, 2018). This is not to say we do not have expertise, though it remains interesting as to what we have expertise *in*.

We remain embedded in the traditions and practices of our theoretical backgrounds, our analytic families in which we have invested so much. Such a world contrasts with patients who, as with addiction in many cases, insist on pathologizing pain (Stolorow, 2016) and fallibility, resistant to an empathic recognition they have reason to distrust yet subtly crave, the latter all but confirming their "neediness."

Patients from addictive worlds are often profoundly unfamiliar with the perception and speaking of emotion directly, a natural-sounding game (to us), that most primitive of recognition, embedded for many in the traumatic stickiness of coercion and mind-reading: an omniscience coercively, compulsively demanded. "Isn't that obvious?" Jonathan once said, when I asked about his feelings. "No," I said, and he laughed with surprise.

Such disjunctive tension can overshadow micro-tendrils of forward edge seeking (Tolpin, 2009). In fact, it is developmental for most simply to cross our threshold. It was also admirably risky of Jonathan to express his anger toward me, a chance to feel fully alive.

The shame of his need (disavowed yet perseverant) led to his cycles of erotic enactment, which then perpetuated shame; one cannot remove such desires by "surgery", any more than we can fully step outside our perspective.

He was thus blind to what drove him in repetition, his affective depths unilluminated, the most foreign language game of all.

In fact, his mother had abandoned the family when he was two, his residual anger toward this abandonment seen as his "failing" due to her reactive pushback. Later, he found safety in booze and isolation, shielding himself from his own "inner parent," benumbing the human contact he shamefully yearned for.

In other words, he lacked the means of playing a game of intimate spokenness, stuck in confused self-loathing, when the orgasm faded and intimacy with women began. Their anger at him was painful yet expected.

Thus, a retreat to the intrapsychic, an inexpressibly safe exile, in the certainties of his recovery slogans, where the problem is always in the mirror, statements both protective and imprisoning (Brandchaft, 2010). My own analytic entrapment there spoke instructively (if silently) of our dilemma.

We can know how to define "love," "fear," and "desire," without knowing what they mean to individuals. I remember the director of a program for porn addiction, who told me he aimed to supplant lust with intimacy. He said this casually, as if it were truly a matter of learning a definition.

"All life is encounter," as Buber (1970, p. 61) put it. We know such processes historically but not presently, such uncertainty possibly provoking anxiety, due perhaps to our asymmetrical dependence on patients, an acknowledgment of co-embedded existence.

Perhaps knowledge in the analytic sense is closer to *wisdom*, a disciplined intuition, a matter of knowing what I do not yet know but want or need to know, in order to help the one before me. There is often the temptation to compulsively name such processes, as if they are constituted by words alone. It remains surprisingly easy to confuse content with its framing, just as with any substance or behavior and the voids they attempt to fill.

References

Bollas, C. (2018). *The shadow of the object: Psychoanalysis of the unthought known*. Routledge. Originally published 1987.

Brandchaft, B. (2010). *Towards an emancipatory psychoanalysis: Brandchaft intersubjective vision* (B. Brandchaft, S. Doctors, & D. Sorter, Eds.) Routledge.

Buber, M. (1970). *I and thou* (W.A. Kaufmann, Trans.) Scribner.

Freud, S. (1917). Mourning and melancholia. In J. Strachey (Ed. & Trans.), *The standard edition of the complete psychological works of Sigmund Freud* (Vol. 14, pp. 237–258). Hogarth Press.

Haber, D. (2022, March 3). Medusa moments in psychoanalysis. Blog of the APA. Retrieved from https://blog.apaonline.org/2022/03/03/medusa-moments-in-psychoanalysis

Hatab, L. (2017). *Proto-phenomenology and the nature of language: Dwelling in speech I*. New Heidegger Research (series). Roman & Littlefield.

Heaton, J. (2013). *The talking cure: Wittgenstein on language as bewitchment & clarity*. Palgrave Macmillan. Originally published 2010.

Jones, D.B. (2009). Addiction and pathological accommodation: An intersubjective look at impediments to the utilization of alcoholics anonymous. *International Journal of Psychoanalytic Self Psychology*, 4(2):212–234. https://doi.org/10.1080/15551020902738250

Orange, D.M. (2014). And we shall be changed: To hold theory lightly is to surrender assumptions: Discussion of clinical narrative by Steven Stern. *International Journal of Psychoanalytic Self Psychology*, 9(3):193–199. https://doi.org/10.1080/15551024.2014.917459

Stolorow, R.D. (2015). A phenomenological-contextual, existential, and ethical perspective on emotional trauma. *The Psychoanalytic Review*, 102(1):123–138. https://doi.org/10.1521/prev.2015.102.1.123

Stolorow, R.D. (2016). Pain is not pathology. *Existential Analysis*, 27(1):70–74.

Tolpin, M. (2009). A new direction for psychoanalysis: In search of a transference of health. *International Journal of Psychoanalytic Self Psychology*, 4(sup1):31–43. https://doi.org/10.1080/15551020902958643

Wittgenstein, L. (1969). *On certainty* (D. Paul, & G.E.M. Anscombe, Trans.) (G.E.M. Anscombe, & G.H. Von Wright, Eds.) Basil Blackwell.

Wittgenstein, L. (2009). *Philosophical investigations* (4th ed.) (G.E.M. Anscombe, P.M.S. Hacker, & J. Schulte, Trans.) (P.M.S. Hacker, & J. Schulte, Eds.) Blackwell Publishing Ltd. Originally published 1953.

3 Dissociation and Bewitchment in Analytic Dialogue

Having a Word

"So," he said at the top of the analytic hour, "where should we start?" He looked at me expectantly, with a bit of a chuckle. Anxiety, perhaps, or bemusement?

He's holding out, I thought, determined to upend this tedious chess match, which had us stalemated.

This was a recurring theme with Jeremy, a pleasant but rigidly organized patient in his mid-30s, who sought my help in finding a partner. He was stuck there, at the starting line of his life—and soon so were we.

Jeremy had trouble starting new ventures; he wanted a new job but feared that it (or he) would not measure up. The same went for finding a boyfriend. Identifying as bisexual, he had decided to pursue men, though anything beyond a fling was difficult to imagine, let alone sustain. What if he were rejected by someone he really liked, and ended up stuck with someone he hated?

Jeremy grew up an only child in a Midwestern suburb that was tolerant yet still heteronormative. He found sexuality confusing and shameful, as with so many of his developmental desires, including in a social life with his straight-edge friends who were viewed as "troublemakers" by his helicoptering mother. His mother endlessly overstepped, with Dad uninterested in anything besides his work. Jeremy related this to me with a bemused detachment, with flashes of a simmering cauldron he dared not express.

His parents constantly, bitterly fought, divorcing when Jeremy hit puberty ("ten years too late," he quipped). His workaholic dad left the house and his son's life, Jeremy now coerced into a surrogate partner/caregiver role for a mother often bedridden due to chronic illness, with (he suspected) a growing dependence on painkillers. When her prescriptions ran out early, she became rageful. He now related to me how hard this was … for *her*.

Jeremy's mother kept him on a tight leash well into his teen years. Yet I too soon chafed against the constraints of Jeremy's detours, as if he were awaiting me to fill the gaps, peer into his own mind. He often apologized for being "a difficult patient."

DOI: 10.4324/9781003598534-3

There were flashes of Jeremy's wounded anger toward his mother's rage and father's absence, followed by a silencing guilt, at which point our dialogue skidded to a halt.

The atmosphere was suffocating at times. Affectivity of almost any kind was intolerable for him, intensity fast neutered by jokes or diversions. He once asked if he won the award for most difficult patient. "I imagine what you've lived through is difficult," I said. "That's the self-centered view," he responded, as if it were immoral to recognize his own suffering.

Affectivity became akin to original sin. Was I the snake in his Garden of Dissociative Eden? Either way I couldn't win; he heard my curiosity as criticism.

Forget being on the same page; we weren't even in the same *book*.

What puzzled me most was not Jeremy's reluctance to speak, but our shared conviction that the right words—if only we could find them—would somehow break the stalemate.

Accommodation and Dissociation

Like many patients, Jeremy arrived hoping to be more accommodating at work, less irritated with inept superiors and his mother—banishing the anger that quickly turned into guilt. Even now he walked on eggshells with her.

He also admitted he was well defended with me: "I'm a black belt, you've met your match," he said, again with a chuckle that annoyed me, as if he took pride in the self-defense that kept him imprisoned (I suppose it was safe there).

"Do I *want* to change?" he would ask himself at times, followed by long pauses. It seemed at such moments that it was up to me to persuade him of the benefits of change (of my efficacy?), with him on the sidelines, arms crossed with skepticism. My attempts to understand *this* dynamic were ineffective, given his reactive self-blame, which alternated with a subtle, intellectualized superiority.

Often at the start of sessions, he would ask what threads to pull on that day; he was accustomed to accommodating, and now I was to accommodate in turn. Expressed curiosity about my part in this, after nearly a year of treatment, again sent us in circles. "I don't know why I don't know what to talk about," he'd say, grinning nervously. "I was hoping you could tell me, though I suppose that's 'against the rules.' I guess nothing feels all that … urgent?"

Then, the bemused chuckle.

At times I reintroduced a previous thread, where he often became impatient: "This doesn't have juice this week," he would say. While my goal was to open emotional windows for ventilation, his was to keep them locked (while complaining less).

Jeremy was extremely bright and often humorously engaging, while also organizing nearly all life activities (including therapy) into "checklists." "Just gimme the boxes to check and I'm a happy camper," he would say. (I had no such boxes to offer.)

It all worked well for him, often enough. He managed a local chain of juice shops and "ran a tight ship." He was kind to employees but very hardworking. Even a drop of frustration toward a fumbling employee or clueless supervisor, sounding mild to me, resulted in surges of guilt.

I observed that his agentic moves were framed mechanically, ever calculated; he agreed with that observation but couldn't imagine an alternative. When he said he hoped to "nail down the dating issues," this too was ticking a box, while recognizing this was "probably the wrong approach."

He was loath to discuss his binge drinking and overeating, but he did reluctantly acknowledge these, occasionally. To me it made sense, given that so much of his emotionality was on lockdown; these binges were like prison escapes. Yet this topic too was foreclosed, as these shameful binges (the spirit escaping from its cell) should have ended long ago. "What's the fix?" he asked, with an ironic smile, like a riddle whose answer confounded me.

Bewitchment by Language

I noticed we repeated the same phrases and rituals week to week—at the start, especially. *How was the week, Jeremy? Did they replace that inept delivery guy yet?* I found myself hoping the right remark or comment from me might shake things loose. "Your boss sounds a bit Mom-ish," I would say. "It all comes back to blaming Mom, eh?" he would say, with a knowing tone. I explained why I made that connection, hinting at more visceral explorations—though this too was given to rational sorting. *How*, he would ask, *can one be more visceral*?

We both somehow believed that the "correct words" would set us free, a symptom of what Wittgenstein (2009) refers to as the "bewitchment of our intelligence by means of language" (§ 109), discussed throughout this book.

Wittgenstein reminds us that everyday speech does not represent reality like a photograph; it expresses a perspective on experience—the stories we invent. Because we are the frame through which we see the world, the frame itself usually goes unnoticed. In therapy, another person can begin to make it visible.

Therapy helps make this frame visible by developing language games through which experience can be reflected upon. How has the patient come to see things in this or that way? With Jeremy such questions put him on the back foot. My observing he saw things a certain way almost always implied such a way was "wrong", setting us again in opposition.

When Jeremy spoke of his "failures" at dating, he described *being* a failure—a direct equivalence, bypassing the underlying aim of his pursuits, the guilty verdict ever hovering (like his mother's skepticism and father's nonpresence). The construction of such a viewpoint was also unseen: a dimly befogged windshield through which he viewed … everything. The problem is that, in the grammar of the concrete, windshield and vision are fused. The same may subtly hold for our analytic views which, humanly speaking, can be like wearing "a pair of glasses on our nose through which we see whatever we look at. It never occurs to us to take them off" (Wittgenstein, 2009, § 103).

What is revealed in speech is not how "reality" is, but how *we are*. Dissociated patients often see things concretely, as if their words *directly* portray how the world is: concretization versus metaphor. Such use bypasses any notions of framing, personalized speech, or (most pertinently) the *value* of such personalization, of speaking a world of one's own.

When underlying affectivity is deflected or avoided (and Jeremy and I both contributed), reflective space collapses. Participants end up awaiting the *Godot* (Beckett, 1982) of some magical statement or insight, as if words alone are transformative, rather than a spoken *practice* allowing the patient to more dynamically express his lived emotionality.

The main vehicle for change, I believe, is the relationship itself and the dialogue it manifests in the consulting room: the enacted emergence of new grammars.

So how did we end up repeating the same tired lines over and over, as if saying them louder, or with minor variance, might finally do the job?

Mutual Anxiety

We tend to underestimate the power of the unspoken affect organizing our viewpoint, driven by unnamed feelings, fears, and hunger that may appear irrational or threatening to the conscious status quo. Our dreams reveal to us our demands and terrors, as do our sudden rages on the road, along with our private longings and reveries, our shared bursts of laughter, or unsettling *angst,* signs of an unnamed influence: a key idea starting with Freud.

Enigmatic anxieties befog perspective, provoking binaries: either/or grammars in which words become thing-like, pawns on the board. A transactional relatedness emerges, drained of pulse.

For Jeremy, this meant a pensive silence I had trouble tolerating; he seemed terrified he was failing me, which my spoken curiosity confirmed. It came to mean something was off—leading to the trap of explanation. Generally, however, dialogue *shows* but does not *explain* psychic dynamics. These shifts of perspective are impossible to formulize; that they happen at all may be testament to the power of human speech. We start to *hear* a word differently, spoken in a different key. Perhaps this word is our new response to the familiar: unexpectedly jolting. Sometimes therapists and analysts notice their different uses of the same or similar terms. It dawns on the patient that "love" may not mean "obey," that a patient's resistance is actually a lack of familiarity with what we seem to be implying (i.e., that there is a possibly sabotaging "something" behind their sentences).

For the most part Jeremy remained sheltered in rational bewitchment, ready with the right idea or phrase to detour pain; *it wasn't so bad, I'm doing pretty well, there are people starving in India*—moves so familiar he no longer thought about them. But such arid safety carries a cost, he started to notice, including his isolation and ceaseless inner monologues of doubt: a subjectivity still shaken by his mother's volatility and demands. This became the unseen backdrop of his world, painful and brutish.

Inflexibly rational speech becomes a numbing chain of words: labyrinths leading nowhere. I think I missed a chance to grab the golden thread when I heard his complaints about "dead-end topics," as he was protesting neglect on my part for answering *for* him, a bit too quickly. There was something else I was missing.

In fact, our stalemate lay in the game we described rather than played. Analytic life is *lived,* not explained or "figured out." Figuring out *follows* the enactment of affect, thunder after lightning—as when we ask, "what just happened?"

Language is always catching up. The bolt of affect Jeremy flashed was not aimed at me, but at the speaker who was jeopardizing the relationship by needing help, frustrated he could not think his way through the relational labyrinth alone: a rigged game, and not in his favor, even if it remained the only one he knew.

"Believe Me": A New Game

One day I said to Jeremy, during a tense exchange about his struggle to get sessions started, "It's like you're deep in a fortress when we begin, I can't reach you, and I don't know why."

"And when you ask why and I say I *don't know*," he responded, subtly exasperated, "it's like you don't believe me." There was actual distress here; I *heard it:* injury rather than strategy.

He said, "It's like I … lack the vocabulary."

I sat up in my chair. Of course he did, because he *didn't know the language game!*

I had been treating his "I don't know" as resistance when it was closer to a kind of homelessness. Emotional exchange does not function like a vocabulary to be memorized; it belongs to a *practice* of recognition between people.

I hadn't recognized it either, because any such game is *mutually* defined, one I inherently assumed he knew (but refused to play). Thus we were locked in a shadow battle over who made the rules. Even when he deferred to me, he responded with protest because my rules sounded threatening—or rather, foreign. He did not know them and could not play them, *and could not say so,* as this only, shamefully, reiterated his inadequacy. After all I was speaking plain English.

In fact his "I don't know" made *me* anxious, as if he were warily sidestepping the question, keeping me on the outside rather than revealing his own alienation. *C'mon man, get with it.* I needed, again, to "dumb it down," for both of us; he was inhabiting the grammar of his constriction, as was I by default, the difference being that it was as familiar to him as the wallpaper.

What we needed here, in a way, was less chess and more Go Fish.

In fact Jeremy had never been allowed to *literally* play much—to be a kid among kids, even before his parents' divorce. (I imagine he came out of the womb reading a book.) Emotional spontaneity was discouraged or ignored; precocity kept the peace, in his avoiding saying "ouch" as an imposition. He didn't even know the purpose of its utterance, although "ouch" was at the root of the very language game I was trying to initiate—for him a foreign dialect.

Some patients assume that recognizing emotion simply means naming it, as though words were labels rather than moves in a mutual game, like affixing a label, as if the label itself transforms. This is why concretizing patients (such as this one) often say, "So I realize I'm anxious, now what?" They have made the essential move; bewitchment stands its ground.

What enlivens these forms of life (Wittgenstein, 2009) is responsiveness and recognition. The child is encouraged to say "ouch" via a confirming response, not to "report" but to *relate* a sensation of pain or physical distress in need of soothing. The arrival of soothing confirms the value of expression. These primal, tender words carry the currency of recognition, value on the dollar of speech, like a parent learning to discern their baby's cries. Such cries or other expressions are devalued when a caregiver's needs take precedence. Here the ground of relatedness falters, and the infant learns that its cries are "problematic" for others. (How many times did Jeremy say he was a difficult patient?)

It isn't a matter of *knowing* or reciting feeling words but of understanding *their purpose* and use, in an atmosphere of recognition: the practices of coexistence.

I often contributed to our stalemate by "explaining" how this all worked, and why affect was important, inviting more fraught and empty chatter. But we cannot explain the *value* of recognition; we do our best to embody it, hitting dead ends while committed to banging on (as the Brits say), with as much empathic frankness as possible.

Why did it take so long to get this?

Throwing Away the Book: A Shameful Memory

Jeremy was so self-critical that I feared my frustration would cause even more shame, as with his mother, a caution related to my own early experience, including an imperative to speak with undue caution to deeply insecure caregivers.

Jeremy had been traumatized by a mother which reminded me in many ways of my own childhood; I too had a parent who shut me down when threatened.

When I was in middle school, I borrowed a book from the library on alcoholic families, amazed that such a book even existed. I left it in the living room one evening, and my father spotted it the next morning on the coffee table. He whitened with rage, furiously whispering for me to *get that goddamn book outta here.* I duly, shamefully obeyed.

Words now felt darkly powerful in their capacity to harm others and push them away—the book like a tome from Voldemort's library.

This is why I misheard Jeremy's "I don't know" as dismissive, somewhat, akin to "get that question outta here!" In fact Jeremy was protecting *me* from his "burdensome" need for expanded understanding. What I missed was the despair befogged by words, shamed by the sin of not knowing, both of us quietly living in it.

Jeremy too had been taught that honest self-expression is threatening and thus *verboten.* We remained in the grip of a fear of overexposure, of *any* exposure, hiding behind concepts.

Still we kept at it, and in doing so I showed Jeremy over time that he was not "too difficult" for me, disconfirming his worst fear (abandonment), even if he lacked the vocabulary—the relational "permission" and experience—to play a more intimate game.

I told Jeremy that this "vocabulary," in his illuminating statement, was simpler than we were presuming. Perhaps all we needed was a way for me to help him say, or understand what was scary about saying, in his own words, "His absence hurt and pissed me off" or "Why was Mom such a bitch sometimes?" and "but I feel like shit in saying that."

Eventually he was able to express hurt and fury at his mother, and father, with the remorse that followed, *as if he were killing her*. Perhaps because these were not interpretations but utterances he had never been allowed to make.

Often the languaging of the problem reveals the problem. An addicted patient describes the frustration of not being able to "figure out" how to control drinking *or the craving to do so*, a frustration leading again to the bottle. A new language game is needed entirely, one speaking to and of psychic or soulful suffering.

Consider the term "dissociation." "Dissociated affect" indicates *something* pushed aside or disavowed, like a child exiled into hiding. But that *something* eludes definition, giving it a hazy quality, it tempts us to see it … like a child in hiding—that is, quasi-literally.

I got stuck ruminating on *what* was being dissociated, as if naming it alone were restorative. But what matters is not just *what* is dissociated, but what *purpose* is served by the evasion (usually a fundamental safety). We can get caught up in the *what* and become dissociated ourselves! The (unseen) pushing away is as important as "what" is disavowed: an unspoken no-thing until it enters the something-ness of analytic dialogue.

Here we are called to dwell in what Wilfred Bion, citing John Keats, called "negative capability" (in Grotstein, 2024, p. 109): the uneasy acceptance of not knowing, despite our being seen as experts, while committed to listening and observing as closely as possible. Our expertise is paradoxical: much of it consists of making space for what is not yet expressible.

When we sense a well-defended patient's unnamed affective stirrings, we may feel pushed away—exiled from language, in a sense, though our job is, presumably, one of *knowing what to say*.

This negation of rawly spoken emotionality has become habitual for so many patients—enacted detours compulsively repeated. This void-like presence—the aversion of nearly any "blip" of affect—becomes a Balaska-like limit (see Introduction), one calling for clinical creativity.

Silence is often safety, under an authoritarian regime, whether that regime is political or psychical. It also takes time to see how this works for *this* patient, to fill the chasm of silence with curiosity and desire for authentic speech in the face of such stubborn inarticulation. And so the work remains difficult. As Bion suggested, patient and analyst develop a means of communication *while communicating*—drawing the map as they go (in Reiner, 2012).

But one cannot explore the terrain via a map alone, as if trying to describe a city via a ground plan. Relationships are like cities visited, explored, mapped from *within*, not above (the language game initiated by traumatizing environments).

The analyst, too, must occasionally set aside their theoretical "map," banished from the lush gardens of familiarity and into the desert of unspeakability, terrain more aridly foreboding than our case studies often indicate. Seedlings of new language games arrive through practice and trial and error, taking root in the *something* of expressions finally heard.

References

Beckett, S. (1982). *Waiting for Godot*. Grove Press. Originally published 1954.

Grotstein, J. (2024). *A beam of intense darkness: Wilfred Bion's Legacy to Psychoanalysis*. Routledge. Originally published by Karnac in 2007.

Reiner, A. (2012). *Bion and being: Passion and the creative mind.* Karnac Books.

Wittgenstein, L. (2009). *Philosophical investigations* (4th ed.) (G.E.M. Anscombe, P.M.S. Hacker, & J. Schulte, Trans.) (P.M.S. Hacker, & J. Schulte, Eds.) Blackwell Publishing Ltd. Originally published 1953.

4 Maria Balaska on Wittgenstein, Lacan, and the Limits of Language

Beyond the Limit

Beyond the Limit: Interview with Maria Balaska

I recently had the pleasure of conversing with philosopher Maria Balaska about language, meaning, and her book, *Wittgenstein and Lacan at the Limit: Meaning and Astonishment* (Balaska, 2019).

Balaska engagingly discusses how Wittgenstein and Lacan, two thinkers intensely preoccupied with our life with (and within) language, approach the difficulty of making philosophical sense of moments of wonder and astonishment. Each thinker approaches the problem from different yet oddly resonant angles, moments of what Balaska calls groundlessness. The book is a dense but clearly described journey into the question of how to make sense of such ungrounded wonder, which departs from the logical grounding of our world (in Wittgenstein's case) or meaning that is freed from the usual chain of signifiers (in Lacan's).

Wittgenstein offers the example, in his *Lecture on Ethics* (1993), of experiencing wonder at the existence of the world. This is in the context of what he calls relative value versus absolute value, astonishment at existence in the latter category. The forms of language offer us only the former, Wittgenstein believed. To say in amazement that "the world exists"—to which one might remark, "well, of course it does!"—observes nothing new about the world, no new facts. Yet the world at such moments appears as good, of unquestionable value, via (in this fleeting moment) its expansive *thereness*.

For Wittgenstein this "goodness" exists beyond the logical, in the realm of the ethical or aesthetic (in what counts as goodness in our conduct, or how we discern goodness, respectively), neither of which is factual nor rationally arguable, or directly observable: it is inferred, as with the psychological. One cannot argue (logically) for an ethical perspective.

Thus our wonder at the world, its transcendent goodness (or wholeness), refers to … some ineffable "inner sensation"? Is it all just "in our mind," a hallucination or briefly delectable psychosis? Is *our* sense of wonder something another mind cannot really grasp?

DOI: 10.4324/9781003598534-4

Wittgenstein, at this stage of his thinking (his early, Tractarian period), insists our words are

> vessels capable only of containing and conveying….natural [i.e., factual] meaning and sense. … Ethics, if it is anything, is supernatural and our words will only express facts; as a teacup will only hold a teacup full of water even if I were to pour out a gallon over it.
>
> (1993, p. 40)

Astonishment on this view is disconnected from the rationally evident; our cup runneth over. Wittgenstein is certain that "if we wish to understand and unravel what has created this astonishment in us, we are doomed to fail" (Balaska, 2019, p. 21). We might try to establish some cause and effect or other schematic, but this is weak tea. Wonder is groundless, beyond logical foundation, in that a "set of facts [about the world's existence] comes to have an absolute significance for the person who is astonished" (p. 19).

Thus, Balaska asks, are there "ways to express the astonishment in language without a sense of constraint [or qualification]? And, if so, what is the merit of that expression?" (p. 27). How, in other words, does one establish via language the significance of astonishment or transcendence, given language's shallow (absolutist) cup?

Wittgenstein's Lecture—his only public remarks, incidentally—were given shortly after the publication of the *Tractatus Logico-Philosophicus* (2013). He does not disparage ethics; quite the contrary. He is after our situatedness within language, following the *Tractatus*' famous pronouncement that "the limits of my language mean the limits of my world" (§ 5.6). For Wittgenstein, ethics (and the aesthetic or, again, what counts as valuable or worthy) lies beyond the limits of the logical or rationally founded, which Balaska argues remain value free … just *there*.

There is often tension in Wittgenstein's work, between what must be *shown* versus merely said or explained (as in what storytelling *shows* us about our condition, which Balaska discusses via a passage from Dostoevsky).

As Balaska puts it, "Logic pervades the world; the limits of the world are also its limits" (2019, p. 184). One cannot argue syllogistically for being a vegetarian or being sober in a recovery program, or practicing psychoanalysis. One lives a certain way, and in doing so reflects its value to an inferring other. Such value is unlike that of a propositional fact, such as "today is Tuesday." (Though today, even such basic propositions are increasingly contested.)

It is easy to believe value or commitment has metaphysical qualities: we are tempted to believe it, a notion Wittgenstein protested throughout his work. We may use science to "prove" the workings of nature or the human body or brain, but these are merely factual statements, just "what is." "We have to waken to wonder," Wittgenstein said, "science has a way of putting us to sleep again" (in Bearn, 1997, p. ii). In fact Wittgenstein (1993) suggests it is a mistake to attempt to find the miraculous via the employment of language, when the miracle is the existence of language itself.

Wittgenstein's *Tractatus*, which I will briefly describe (key to the discussion below), provides a still-provocative, dense overview of how the logical workings of language, our propositional facts, or facts-about-things (the basic properties of the things in the world), make up our view of the world and its expectant workings. This is sometimes referred to as Wittgenstein's picture theory.

Propositional facts collectively correspond to the facts about the things of the world, or "all that is the case" (Wittgenstein, 2013, § 1)—for example, gravity pulls objects to the ground, the sun rises in the east, and a chair is typically used for sitting. These are facts, revealing nothing about how to live purposefully or ethically. They are simply there (as with mathematical logic, where 2 + 2 = 4).

Moments of astonishment (benevolent calamity) break through and perturb our everyday rationality and assumptions, the expectedness of our lives, as "the question of individuation arises with one's contact with the groundlessness of meaning; hence, the experience of astonishment is a potential entry point to it" (Balaska, 2019, p. 186).

Yet for an analytic patient, groundlessness might be terrifying, appearing as dread or terror (as Balaska illustrates). I wonder if our apparent groundedness is what proves illusory in the end: another of Stolorow's (2007) tranquilizing absolutes, as wonder at the world serves as a more benign intrusion. It seems you cannot have one without the other.

All of this is pertinent for the analytic process, as participants seek to develop mutually understandable terms and concepts. Competing glossaries lead to confusion, though we often think of our glossary as the correct one, upon which our conceptual schemas rest. Yet many patients with low self-esteem blur factual or logical forms with depressive inference; that is, "I cannot achieve a good result, and am therefore not good" or "only top grades or salary establish my worth," and so on. "Good" becomes a tyrannical signifier, and *fact*.

Balaska also interweaves Lacan into her discussion, who "takes the problem of groundlessness to run across all kinds of human discourse" (2019, p. 41). This includes the idea of our inherited world of signifiers: an as-yet unspoken sense of the Real, or swirl of experience difficult to symbolize (such as floating anxiety, traumatic overwhelm, and so on): a form of Donnell Stern's (2010) unformulated experience, albeit resistant to formulation. As Balaska puts it,

Meaning is never ours to make, and believing that it is (ours to make) belongs to (what Lacan calls) an imaginary position, a fantasy that we can control what (our) words mean, not unlike when Humpty Dumpty says that his words mean whatever he wants… (Balaska, 2019, p. 42).

This dilemma lies here, in the unsymbolized Real, per Lacan, or in "essential nonsensicality" per Wittgenstein (in Balaska, 2019, p. 32)—evasive to language yet powerfully present (see the overflowing teacup above). Such moments call for us to become "creatively involved in meaning" (p. 46), reminiscent of the clinical creativity required of dyadic participants in needing to "manufacture means of communication *while communicating*" (Bion, 1975, p. 31, my italics).

In this sense our imagination and creativity become midwives to more personalized expression, as the ethical exists beyond the limit of language's normative parameters.

Balaska suggests we lean into these barriers, into the inexpressible, to tango with the Real, for it is when we respond "with a reflective involvement with meaning *that the ethical character of these experiences emerges*" (2019, p. 204, my italics). We are then spontaneously inventing new forms of living and signifying (in analysis and elsewhere), in our spoken co-existence, the dance of meaning-making.

I hope you will enjoy our conversation. I thank Maria for her generous cooperation and wonderful book, whose rereading continues to reward.

Darren: Hi, good morning—or afternoon.

Maria: Hello!

Darren: Are you in England?

Maria: Yes, I'm in London.

Darren: Great city, I miss it. So to get the discussion going, did you start off doing counseling work before moving to academia?

Maria: I started off as a psychologist, training as a psychotherapist. I worked with adults and children for a few years, and then I decided to do a PhD in philosophy. But in some other sense, philosophy was already there when I was younger, during my BA studying. When I was a teenager, I already knew some of Wittgenstein's work, and I was interested in his ideas. So it felt natural for me to go from being a psychologist to doing work on Wittgenstein, and it still feels like that. It feels like the two disciplines have a lot in common, yeah?

Darren: For sure. I'm quite interested in the parallel between therapy to Wittgenstein and philosophy. What do you see as the overlap?

Maria: I guess it depends on what one wants to do with these disciplines. For me, a big part was always that I want to understand the human being. I'm just intrigued by this, and psychoanalysis in particular, which was the discipline that

I was most interested in when I was doing clinical work, which very much looks at the human as a whole. Philosophy does the same in different ways, but I see them as complementary. It's like one zooms in and the other zooms out.

In terms of Wittgenstein in particular, well as you yourself know, he's much stricter with the concepts, as he looks for clarity, something that I think psychotherapy in a way does not, and maybe we should not blame them, because that's not their focus.

Darren: But it's an interesting idea. I mean, it is a focus for me and some of my colleagues.

Maria: It is important, because otherwise you end up with a confused understanding of "the psyche" that you then impose on your patients or clients. So I think it's essential to have or seek to have *some* philosophical clarity when you work with concepts like "the unconscious" and so on.

Darren: I wonder if you had an example there, like the opposite of Wittgenstein's "perspicuity," where it gets fuzzy in psychology and maybe confusing. It's a tricky question.

Maria: Perhaps the example I have is not so much a case of clarity as a case of not having refined your understanding of the human being enough … but if you have a limited version or limited account of what "happiness" in human life is about, or what's available or possible in terms of how one can be happy, or what it *means* to be happy, then you may be working in a direction that is problematic, either because it is too naive and unrealistic or because it is too shallow.

I'm mostly thinking here of a more superficial or unquestioning understanding of what it means to live a good human life.

Darren: Well some patients read, with all due respect, or consume … how to say it … mainstream articles about how to be happy, and then this is the concept they're bringing in. "I want to be my best self" or "live my best life," and so on. But what this means is unclear.

Maria: Yes. And within psychoanalysis, you have this problem in terms of a lack of an account of the ethical, which starts from Freud's limited understanding of ethics as reducible to cultural norms and the Superego. So this is an example of how a more sophisticated conception of the human life as what is drawn toward goodness can be helpful to psychoanalysis.

Another more Wittgenstein-inspired example of how philosophy can be of help to psychoanalysis is the conceptual clarity that it brings, and there are many concepts in psychoanalysis that would benefit from it. For example, think of the concept of the unconscious, like when you speak about what the unconscious drives you to do. This has such far-reaching consequences for how we understand our motives and responsibility.

Darren: It's interesting, sometimes people say, just in general practice, "Maybe I unconsciously meant to do this." What does that mean?

Maria: Yes, exactly. What does that mean?

If you take away the word "unconsciously" there, what happens? What does it add? What happens if you don't have that word there? Yes, I think that's the kind of question that Wittgenstein would ask.

Darren: There is an interesting book by David Archard (2024) that discusses this topic by the way, I recommend it. Now, I have a possibly strange question. And I want to get to your book after this. But Wittgenstein read Freud, and had very mixed reactions. He recognized Freud's genius and his powerful way of thinking. But he also took issue with some of his more positivist conclusions. And I often wonder if some of the more contemporary approaches to psychoanalysis, where … and I hope this isn't too idealistic … but basically you have two participants trying to co-create a language game in some mutually understandable way. Intersubjective thinkers talk about the hermeneutics of dialogue. I ask myself if Wittgenstein might have some appreciation of this as a co-constructed world or context, or would he remain skeptical? My secret hope is he would say, "Okay, this is a little more like it."

Maria: I agree. I think the idea of therapy as conversation would be much closer to how Wittgenstein sees it. More like a *practice,* or a way of relating, rather than just a theory.

Darren: And not an abstract metaphysical theory or metapsychological theory. Okay. So your book, and what really got me thinking, where I became preoccupied, is with the idea of the limit, the limit of what we can say to describe what we're experiencing, in the case of something like wonder or astonishment. We live within those limits. And once I read the book and started thinking about the limit, it's there, almost always. We seem to *live* the limit. It's a little hard to explain, but we're always at the limit, in a sense, in our life, in our dialog with other people.

So I'm curious about the genesis of the book. It was very interesting how you settled on the *Tractatus*.

Maria: Well your mention of the limit does link to the choice of the *Tractatus*, which is I think the obvious place in Wittgenstein to go to, if you're looking to think about limits. What I find interesting about the concept which, as you say, if you start thinking about it, you see it everywhere, or it seems to be a big part of human life, is that it comes with two meanings, or two pictures. One is the picture where you have a limit as an external boundary. So we say, for example, my "patience has reached its limits." And what you mean there is that the patience is almost over, and then some other affect will take its place.

But then you have this other pictorial representation of a limit as an *internal* impossibility, not an external boundary. We can also find an example from the affective life here. Sometimes in relationships, you have limits as … not as the end of the relationship, but as an internal impossibility. Think of the case of certain topics that a couple cannot talk about without the sense that there is something impossible, topics that end up being a no-go zone, without, however, signaling the end of the relationship.

Now in the book, as you know, I'm interested in how the concept of limit appears in our relation to language. And I think one of the main problems that occur when we think of "limits in language" is the first image I mentioned, the picture of a limit as an external boundary, rather than as an internal impossibility or difficulty. When we think of it as an external boundary, then we also think that there is something "beyond language," something that language cannot reach, as it were. Then we give up on words and sense-making, imagine them to be inadequate or powerless. This can have various consequences, philosophical and ordinary. At an everyday level, this can mean abandoning our sense-making capacity and responsibility.

Darren: I see. And there are some interesting passages in your book about that. It's not as if there's some "thing" there that we just can't quite name, right?

Maria: Yes, the temptation or the easy way out is to say "language is not enough." The *Tractatus* is a response to the philosophical version of that temptation. But it's very hard to disconnect life from language, or the human life from language.

Darren: We're embedded in it.

Maria: Exactly.

Darren: So this "something else," would you see it as, well this is where creativity is needed, or imagination, this … I'm going to use a cliché here, but in leaning in or getting creatively involved with our lives.

Maria: Yes, exactly. These limits, or these challenges to sense making that we encounter all the time, not just in philosophy, when we try to make philosophical sense of things, but also in our everyday life, when we try to make sense of who we are, these challenges invite or call for a different kind of involvement with meaning, because a lot of life In language can happen without being involved in sense making. And this might sound strange because I'm obviously talking all the time and communicating and going about things with things. So why? How can one do all that and yet not be involved in sense making? But one can talk and act in ways that are borrowed and unlived. This is what Heidegger calls the *they*, or Cavell likes to think about in terms of convention, and we just rely on these conventions and we can live a life without really being there in our words. I take these cases of limit, where we feel that "I can't find the words," as cases that invite us to become more present as sense-makers, and make language *our* language, and that's exactly where you make something of that experience of limit, and that's the creativity that you referred to and that I discuss in the book.

Darren: I like "make language our language." You also mentioned the *Tractatus* and "the limits of my language are the limits of my world" (2013, § 5.6). Is that what Wittgenstein was talking about? It seems to fit this theme that you're discussing now.

Maria: Yes. I take that as a big part of the *Tractarian* project, to show how impossible it is to be outside language and how the world happens from *within* language.

Darren: And something that I've thought about quite a bit there, about happening within, is Wittgenstein's Lecture on Ethics, which was not long after the *Tractatus* was published. That's a very interesting talk insofar as the limits of ethics or our language of ethics is within the limits of the relative. In both Wittgenstein and Lacan, you're talking about ethics as something developing beyond this limit. I know Lacan is a very different framing, but Wittgenstein seems to say we cannot speak of ethics with philosophical certainty. It's interesting, it would be almost easy to read him as disparaging ethics, but I don't think that's what's going on. So, long story short, I wonder if you could talk about the ethical that's happening in that lecture. I think he says something like, "there are no ethical facts we can speak of" … as if to say, this is something that we have to *live*, not reason. It cannot be metaphysicalized, we cannot logically have some ethical schema, there are limits to how we can discuss it philosophically (pause). It's complicated.

Maria: I guess one question is, if you don't take ethics to be a moral code or a set of tools that you use to solve problems, if you don't do that, and Wittgenstein definitely does not want to think of ethics in that way, because for him that would mean valueless value, the value of ethics must transcend the facts of this world, according to the *Tractarian* structure. All propositions are of equal value, this means all facts are of equal value, there is no value *in* the world of facts (and as he says, if value did exist in the world, it would have no value). And if you want ethics to have that more transcendental aspect to it, then you have to ask the question, how and where does it come from? How am I awakened to a world that is an ethical world, a world where *the good* matters?

It matters in such a way that it can make my world the world of a happy person even if the facts of my world are no different from that of the unhappy person. From the facts themselves alone, you can't get to the Good.

Darren: Is this the ladder he throws away at the end of the *Tractatus*?

Maria: I don't know. The question of the ladder is a rather complicated one in the *Tractatus* scholarship.

Darren: Wittgenstein just gets to the end of the book and says, now we're done, so let's get to the important thing, which we cannot discuss, the most important thing about all this, and disregard the earlier part as nonsense. [ED. NOTE: the actual quote is, "My propositions are elucidatory in this way: he who understands me finally recognizes them as senseless, when he has climbed out through them, on them, over them. (He must so to speak throw away the ladder, once he has climbed up on it)" (2013, § 6.54). There is a great deal of controversy about this quote.]

Maria: I mean he does say [in a letter to a colleague] that the point of the book is ethical, so that's very much in the background of his thinking: ethics, aesthetics, religion, these areas do not fit into a view of language as a set of propositional facts that represent other facts.

Darren: The "facts about things" (2013, § 1) of the world he talks about.

Maria: Yes. So I take the lecture on ethics to be a question about that kind of ethics, and this is where he uses this example of the astonishment at the wonder that the world exists, right?

Darren: Yes, it's beautiful.

Maria: Which has been very important for me and for my thinking, and there he links ethics and language. He says that the miracle of the existence of the world, or that the world exists, can be best expressed as the miracle that language exists. I don't know if I've answered your question.

Darren: Well, I'll tell you what's sticking before we get to Lacan, but this question of "where do we start?" You asked the big question of living the good, or acting upon the good. Where do we start? Is just beyond the limit where we start? Is that what your thought is here, that we start once we get beyond the limit of the sayable?

Maria: I would phrase it as follows: that this kind of ethics may often appear as a limit, as a limit to language. It may often appear as something that I don't know how to express, because when I try to express it, it seems that words fail me. So to go back to the experience he mentions, if I remember this correctly, he takes a walk on a summer's day, and suddenly he's hit by the fact that the world exists. But then, if you try to express that and say to your friend: the world exists!, how are you saying more than the obvious, that the world exists? Of *course* the world exists! So this sense of significance, you don't know where it comes from, and by repeating the same statement, the world exists!, all you do is just state the obvious. But in this difficulty, something important takes place. So I think it's in terms of the expression of profound value, that the limit, or a sense of encountering a limit, arises.

Darren: Of course without that limit, there would be no wonder or astonishment. It's almost baked into the experience, right? And if it's not too much to ask, why wonder versus, and I think I mentioned this in my email to you … as someone who works with a lot of trauma, I myself ask if you see perhaps a continuum spectrum, if that's the right framing, from wonder to dread for example, or perhaps you reach the limit and it's quite frightening. "I have no words for this. I can't …."

Maria: Well, I wrote my second book recently (2024).

Darren: Ah yes, I look forward to reading it.

Maria: It's about anxiety, and a look at how anxiety and wonder, certain forms of them, form an affective pair. How one of them already *contains* the other. But it's also a criticism of a naive distinction between negative and positive feelings. I think a more sophisticated account of the affects of the human can show that it's not that straightforward, that there are negative feelings and over there positive feelings. Very often they are interconnected.

Darren: Yes. I feel Heidegger right next to us on this topic. In fact you gave a nice talk at the BWS (British Wittgenstein Society) on Heidegger and Wittgenstein, which I heard not long ago. And it ties to this, it was a very interesting discussion about anxiety—as opposed to fear, by the way—and then bringing in a Wittgenstein sense of, there's a wonderful phrase you used, "an inarticulate sound." That was quite interesting.

Maria: Thank you. Yes I have worked a lot on this link between Wittgenstein and Heidegger. And an important part of the link is that Wittgenstein had big admiration for Kierkegaard, he read him very seriously. So the link is there, because if he reads Kierkegaard, then Heidegger is not far. And Kierkegaard speaks both about wonder, and about anxiety.

Darren: Yes, and that's a big part of psychoanalytic dialog also. And this is the last quick question before Lacan. There's a lot of tension in the psychoanalytic world around the ethics of various positions. Well, in our whole culture right now, politically and otherwise, but especially in psychoanalytic circles where I travel. It seems like so much of the tension is around coming to terms with what certain words mean. What does "gender affirming" care mean? What do "trans rights" mean? Should we have "DEI" as part of our curriculum? If so, in what capacity? And then arguments or disagreements flare. And sometimes I wonder if philosophy could help there.

Because I think we see a lot of that in our world right now, where basic terms are claimed as defined this way versus that way. And then you have a binary, and it gets very heated. So I guess the question is, do we or can discuss the ethical and come to some kind of agreement?

Maria: It's an interesting question, I don't know how much I can offer here. All I can say is that there's always a tension between the ethical and the political, and the ethics that Wittgenstein proposes in the *Tractatus* highlights more the individual, the personal perspective, rather than the collective. I think someone like Aristotle might be a better place to look at for the connection between living a good life and living a politically engaged life.

Darren: You see this in our culture right now, as in "vaccines work, no they don't."

Maria: It is one thing that links back to a point made earlier, the disconnection of ethics from consequences or outcomes.

Darren: I see what you mean. You're getting away from principles [in focusing on outcomes], the structures or schema of beliefs and values.

Maria: Ethics cannot or must not be reducible to whether there are certain outcomes.

Darren: Yes, this tends to justify the political too often, and we're not agreeing on what, what is the ethical realm, what are the terms or criteria of this conversation, maybe that's what I was trying to say earlier. Okay, so I don't want to leave out Lacan, he'd be quite displeased. What led you to pair the two? You could just have a book on Wittgenstein, but instead, I thought it was an interesting pairing that you brought in Lacan, with both obviously preoccupied with language.

Maria: In a way what led me to pair them is that they are so different, yet they share the focus on language and its central role for the human life. There was also an attempt by Lacan (2007) to say something about the *Tractatus*, which was rather misplaced.

Darren: (laughs) I didn't know that, but it's not surprising.

Maria: Yes, Lacan's arrogance often leads him to a poor analysis of other thinkers. But I think what they have in common is, as you said, the focus on language, but also the idea that how you relate to language has something to do with how fulfilled your life can be. There's something about how we relate to language that links to whether we live a good life.

Darren: Can I just ask you about one quote before we stop? There's a lovely quote on page 209 of your book, "human beings are always already thrown into language determined by signifiers in ways they did not choose, did not anticipate, and usually are not aware of." I just thought that was a very nice encapsulation. The signifier has a great deal of importance in Lacanian theory.

Maria: There are I think two claims made in that passage you just quoted. One is that language matters, that the signifiers we use—the words and the concepts—determine who we are. Again, there's often this problematic idea that language is a set of tools that we use to express our inner life, a life that is already "there" somehow. But this is something radical that Lacan teaches us, that the inner life is already structured in and through signifiers.

So that's one important thing, that we *are* language, or a relation to language. And the other important thing in this quote is the lack of choice. That we are born into the signifiers. I think an easy way to think about this is to think about children and how they come into the world, they're born into a family's history. They are never a *tabula rasa*. They are already… even by having a name and the history of that name, they are already burdened with meanings that they did not choose and that they will have to grow into and try to understand, somethings they will try to get rid of them other times they will try to take ownership of. So, yeah, it's a difficult business.

Darren: You say in the book in several places, be careful about signifiers in isolation. And is that isolation trying to, for lack of a better word, concretize the signifier or control it? I have this sense of almost a unifying definition or uniform concept, as opposed to the relation of signifiers, the broader context of meaning, within which we locate the specific. You discuss the ego a little later on, we don't want the ego to be the controlling element, in trying to occupy the id for instance.

Maria: Yes. And here I'm thinking of this from my clinical work, there are times in our human life where there a word, an affect, a memory is not integrated with the rest of our self-understanding or the other areas of our life. In these cases such signifiers take a special significance, a haunting presence. You must see this very often in your own work.

Darren: Indeed, yes.

Maria: Then what is required is what we call integrating: to bring what haunts us back in relation with other parts of the soul, or other signifiers, and then suddenly it becomes less scary, or it doesn't have the power it has when it is in isolation. It becomes looser and lighter somehow.

Darren: I see. Perhaps in closing you could say something about the creative use of language from a Lacanian point of view. Is it a new chain of signification, or a looser chain, or something loosens? How do we view through a Lacanian lens getting involved with language, what Lacan called I believe *becoming a subject*?

Maria: Lacan, or perhaps it is better to say the literature on Lacan, has two sides: the focus on the Symbolic and desire (usually linked to the first part of his work) and the focus on the Real and on drive (usually linked to the late Lacan). What I see of value in Lacan is the first side. For me, symbolizing and sense-making is all we have. The rest—the limits, the difficulties, the breakdowns—are parts of our individual lives and our socio-political situations, some avoidable, some unavoidable. But in all cases they call for this essential capacity we have: to make sense, to sublimate (to use Lacan's but also Freud's term). This should not be taken as a contrast between some rationalism and the chaos of the Real—I think this is too simplistic. I would speak instead of a lively, creative, courageous stance toward the uncertainties and difficulties, the limits (to go back to where we started) of human life.

Darren: Well, thank you very much, it's been a real pleasure.

Maria: Same. Thank you so much.

References

Archard, D. (2024). *Consciousness and the unconscious* (Psychology Revivals). Routledge: Kindle edition (e-book). Originally published 1984.

Balaska, M. (2019). *Wittgenstein and Lacan at the limit: Meaning and astonishment.* Palgrave Macmillan.

Balaska, M. (2024). *Anxiety and wonder: On being human.* Bloomsbury UK.

Bearn, G. (1997). *Waking to Wonder: Wittgenstein's existential investigations.* State University of New York Press.

Bion, W.R. (1975). *Bion's Brazilian lectures II.* Imago Editora.

Lacan, J. (2007). *The other side of psychoanalysis: Book XVII (Seminar series)* (R. Grigg, Trans.) (J.A. Miller, Ed.) Norton. Originally published 1991.

Stern. D.B. (2010). *Partners in thought: Working with unformulated experience, dissociation, and enactment.* Routledge.

Stolorow, R.D. (2007). *Trauma and human existence.* Routledge.

Wittgenstein, L. (1993). A lecture on ethics. In J. Klagge & A. Nordmann (Eds.), *Philosophical occasions 1912–1951* (pp. 37–44). Hackett Publishing Company.

Wittgenstein, L. (2013). *Tractatus logico-philosophicus.* E-artnow (E-book). Originally published 1922.

5 Either/Or Language Games in Analytic Therapy

Yes or No

The question arrived a few weeks into analytic therapy. Debbie, my bright and endearing 30-something patient, asked me point-blank whether rapper Kendrick Lamar did or did not have a romantic interest in her.

I responded with silence. Was this a joke?

It was not.

Either/or questions—the grammar of binaries—are usually impossible to answer. Life rarely unfolds in black or white. You might have been confronted with yes/no questions in your own life, from a friend, relative, or colleague ("Is mom angry with me – yes or no?" or "Do you think he/she likes me?") and wondered how to respond. Any yes or no answer is bound to be met with an "OK, but …," prolonging a possibly circular exchange.

Debbie and I were, in other words, playing very different *language games*—Wittgenstein's term for the way context shapes how words function. Such context informs the syntax or *grammar* of our speech. Debbie wanted something determinate, while I sensed indeterminate meaning in the thumbs-up or down verdict she sought—like a judgment in the Roman coliseum.

As a psychoanalyst, I attempt to talk with patients about their thoughts and emotions, finding either/or questions difficult to answer (sometimes to the disappointment of patients). Reflecting on Debbie's case led me to consider how binary questions often function less as requests for information than as expressions of anxiety—a search for grounding or reassurance beyond doubt.

Here is Debbie's backstory: Lamar had recently posted on social media about the benefits of sobriety. Debbie, herself clean and sober, "liked" his post and affirmed her own recovery in response. To her amazement, he "liked" her comment. She was even more euphoric when he later posted in support of fans who get "high" on the music rather than substances. How, she asked me, could this not be a covert message or "shout-out" to her? "Or," she asked, "am I crazy?"

I did not think so. But I did sense a hunger for recognition, whose source remained unnamed.

I also found her intelligent and witty, a creative young woman who had suffered unspeakable verbal abuse and "gaslighting" in childhood, from a

DOI: 10.4324/9781003598534-5

narcissistic father ever reminding her he had hoped for a boy. Her mother deferred to him, acting as placatory, often whispering to Debbie: "He doesn't really mean it!"

It was as if Debbie's existence was unreal in her father's eyes, and thus her own (given his systemic position): an invalidation that she had absorbed into her psyche. When a child's psychic injuries are disconfirmed in this way, it creates epistemic trauma, undermining any reliable sense of self or the ability to organize and speak about experience.

The only way her desires could speak, in a way increasingly normative (socioculturally), was through the language of social media, with its likes, retweets, and views. Such like-versus-dislike binaries mirrored the grammar of her early childhood, with expressiveness frozen under the Medusa-like gaze of others. But Lamar appeared to offer a way out: the validation of a global star, a counterspell. But did it really change the game?

I intuited that these early experiences—and their impact on her expressivity—had something to do with our current yes/no dilemma. The slippery ice of the binary was always beneath our feet.

She seemed to hope for me to affirm her take on Lamar's response, myself offering a thumbs-up and dispelling the plaguing self-doubts she had learned to wear like a sweatsuit. What was really at issue was the ever-tenuous nature of her own thoughts and longings.

Online grammar *is* binary but seductive: yes or no, liked or disliked, on point or WTF. One knows where they stand.

But such binaries smoothly mesh, for some patients, with the *archaic* grammar of the either/or: early experiences characterized by neglect or abuse, freezing out the value of more intimate speech. Verdicts are delivered from on high, the child's pain pathologically ignored; later, the patient's spoken desire is itself pathologized, a world of expressivity again circling the drain. Speech in these early worlds becomes disembodied, especially when the threat of getting it "wrong," of deviating from a preapproved script, is unthinkable.

But to submit to the script is equally threatening, as it preserves the psychic kidnapping, with longing numbingly muted.

I frequently observe how anxious or depressed patients are terrified of burdening loved ones (or analysts) with a "neediness" sounding modest to my ears, unspeakably risky for the patient. It is less a melody than a dirge; better to have the online approval of a mega-star.

Debbie seemed destined to fall, in other words, into a "bewitchment of our intelligence by means of language," as Wittgenstein put it in the *Investigations* (2009, § 109). This is his famous caution against holding the meaning of words as universal, transcending all contexts (again, one of the temptations of our slick online interfaces).

Wittgenstein suggested that such confusion arises when language presents us with a misleading picture of how meaning *must* function—an aspect of grammatical hostage-taking, as Debbie's existence was always reducible to a thumbs-up or down. As if she were asking, *Is my desire safe to speak with* you, *Doc?*

Binary language subtly commodifies our psychic forms of life. The thumbs-up becomes fundamental—the grammar of permitted existence, the fragile legitimacy of one's longings. In liking her post, Lamar—a god-like media presence—would confirm her desire to be seen as worthy, redemption once again dependent on the other.

The child wants to be wanted, to hide while knowing others want them found. When such interest is absent, the child feels forgotten in their hiding place. Why live vulnerably when vulnerability has been repeatedly met with indifference? Wittgenstein's "bewitchment" becomes enacted in such scenarios.

Traumatizing systems are shot through with such facticity. The child failed to do X or Y, and therefore *is* contemptible (end of story). In a way, Debbie was testing to see if I too would haughtily reject her "ridiculous" question, the absurdity of needing recognition in some spoken, tangible way: the only language game in town.

A binary question does not merely ask for information; it attempts to stabilize an unstable relational field. The yes/no question itself, when pressed into this role, becomes tyrannical, demanding certainty where lived experience provides ambiguity.

I resisted and even, at times, resented it! I was most interested in what Debbie *felt* about Lamar, what his attention might *mean* to her. But her worldview had been so largely demeaned that "meaning" itself was unipolar, stripped of personal value: the portrait of a hijacked mind.

All such reflection comes with the comfort of hindsight. At the time I often had no clue how to respond. I tend to struggle when a patient asks me to decipher a loved one's thoughts: that is, "Hey Doc, you're a guy….help me understand the male mind. Does my husband *really* want to stay? Will this relationship work?"

Often what the patient is silently seeking is emotional recognition, valuation, or love: "Please tell me I mean something here, *that it's ok for me to want this*." It's a game of spoken absence, sometimes via a telepathy forced upon them in early life, where asking for the explicit deciphering of a system's mixed messages is met with violence and wrath.

Children in alcoholic or misattuned families such as Debbie's are often asked to be psychics.

To help Debbie, I was tempted to also play psychic, read Lamar's tea leaves, "dispel" the uncertainty that terrified her. But therapy is an imperfect process, a dialogue with and not at the patient. Done well, it leads them to confidence in the value of their uniqueness, which cannot really be explained but lived or *shown,* via a trusting relationship, which can feel to a new patient like trusting an unseen net stretched far below the tightrope.

Sometimes the best intervention is stubbornness. I refused to give up on Debbie's emancipation; negotiations continued.

It slowly came to me that I too had been bewitched, thinking that a "yes" would undoubtedly confirm Debbie's worth (good luck with that), while a "no" was tantamount to abandonment. I had been hypnotized by the either/or, as if I had or *should have* an answer from on high. I'd missed the all-important background context: my own anxiety, resulting from an alcoholic upbringing riddled with binaries, especially when it came to the (undoubted) worth of caregivers. Taking a problem to them was raising doubt about their parenting; better for lips to stay zipped.

Finally I said to Debbie, "I think I understand why you're asking. It would be amazing if Lamar really was sending out a coded message. But I can't know that, because I don't know *him,* nor what anyone else is really thinking." She nodded with rational calm. Then I said, "But man, I bet it was *incredible* to get that 'like' from Lamar. His shit is *lit*!"

"Yeah, and he's super hot!" she said, as she burst out laughing. We both started quoting some of his lines (I too am a fan, as is my daughter).

Suddenly, what felt real was her joy and spontaneity, and my not ridiculing the desire her father would have sliced to bits with his razor-like tongue. In fact I observed that celebrities on Instagram were likely *safer than her own family*. Lamar was comfortably distant, would not mock or tear apart her desire to connect—even as such distance also spoke to her conundrum.

From there, we were able to very gradually talk about the contempt and abandonment she had learned to absorb into her own internal dialogues; stepping out of the psychic courtroom run by her father (the hanging judge) was both liberating and risky, with the threat of rearrest, an even harsher sentence.

I acknowledged aloud my own oversight here, my struggle to hear her question, showing her (I hoped) that the "lyrics" of our speech can be heard in different ways, like cover versions of the same song. In this way, aspects of her own father's condemnations shifted over time, not as Truth but as the grandiose self-protections of a deeply insecure man, himself indebted to the scaldingly critical (and misogynistic) language games inherited from *his* father. Such games had cost him; he was now divorced and bitterly alone. Debbie had the opportunity (difficult and grueling) to break the cycle.

The analytic task was, in the end, not to answer the question but to shift the language game in which it seemed to demand a yes or no.

In articulating her abandonment—the grammar of terror and disappointment—she found firmer footing in her dialogues with self and others. A more communal grammar emerged, shared with her analyst, who encouraged what she had long feared to want: to speak a mind of her own.

Reference

Wittgenstein, L. (2009). *Philosophical investigations* (4th ed.) (G.E.M. Anscombe, P.M.S. Hacker, & J. Schulte, Trans.) (P.M.S. Hacker, & J. Schulte, Eds.) Blackwell Publishing Ltd. Originally published 1953.

6 Therapy beyond the Riddle

The Myth of Insight

I often find myself working with extremely intelligent, successful professionals whose careers have stalled or ended due to retirement or illness, or who face an abrupt loss—be it the death or illness of a loved one, or unexpected rupture with a colleague. Many have built their identities around competence, leadership, and decisive thinking; when life suddenly removes the arena in which those traits function, the resulting disorientation can be profound.

Often these go-getters navigate the dilemma using the same intellectual GPS that, unbeknownst to them, helped create it—conceptualizing emotional conflicts as riddles to be solved. Yet the harder they push in this direction, the more the problem seems to return, rolling back down the hill to its original resting place.

Life's disruptions upend our expectations of how things proceed; it's wonderful to come out the other side with insight and renewed purpose, but sweating it out "in the tunnel" is difficult. Isn't there a way to jump the queue?

Many patients are uneasy and unfamiliar with tolerating existential discomfort—what Camus (1983) called *absurdity*, for example, a sudden loss or calamity (or electoral outcome), which requires an extensive "figuring out" in search of a cheat code. These potentially traumatizing changes impact us deeply, altering the contexts or backgrounds of our lives, necessitating new ways of talking, thinking, and living: contingencies of life whose impacts are impossible to circumvent.

This would include an ex-CEO (let's call him Chuck), whom I treated early in my career.

Chuck had been ousted by the board of his successful startup company for two reasons, the first being a maneuvering rival who disliked him (the feeling was mutual), and second, his propensity, by. his own admission, to be "something of an asshole," as he put it. "I don't suffer fools well," he often said. He could also be gentle, compassionate, even humorous (especially with his grandkids), except when disrespected or potentially impeded by an adult. I wondered if some of this was the projection of an inferiority instilled by a commanding father, a military captain.

DOI: 10.4324/9781003598534-6

Chuck was highly driven, only as good as his last achievement (or insight). His ouster from a company he successfully led for many years was a stinging blow. He sought my services because he was bickering with his wife, who harangued him to get help; he had been withdrawn of late, relying on alcohol (and a bit of porn) to soothe his nerves. He resented his wife's harangues, even as he blamed himself for her economic anxiety, due to his failure to find another job as quickly as first expected.

When I initially asked how I might help, he said he hoped to find "aha! moments" to unlock whatever blocked him from rediscovering purpose and vision, while curbing his desire to drink. He was also angry at his father's demand to have more outings together, now that Chuck was unemployed, happy to let his son pick up the tab.

The hope for a decisive insight often assumes that meaning can be secured privately, through an inner recognition that settles the matter once and for all. Yet as Wittgenstein (2009) observed, meaning does not arise in isolation but within shared practices. In the consulting room, understanding emerges less as discovery than as participation in a collaboratively emerging grammar. The possible *aha!* moment is often less a revelation than a new angle on experience hiding in plain view. Often it is the binary phrasing of the riddle—an either/or, wrong/right problem—that obscures its fraught origination (as discussed in the previous chapter).

With Chuck I was reminded of two things: one, that catastrophes—painful and difficult—offer a possible means of renewal, especially in the consulting room: a more engaged participation. Not that it is easy; such jarring shifts reveal our fallibility, humbling or humiliating, undermining our illusions of safety or Stolorow's absolutisms of life (2007). They can also prompt us to explore paths long postponed. (Chuck had a few in mind which sounded promising.)

Secondly, the "aha" thing was a pipe dream. Of course this was never said out loud, but I also never took it seriously—and that was my mistake. Illusions often serve a purpose.

Chuck and I each, in a sense, dismissed each other's language games, whose uses of the word "insight" bore little family resemblance to one another. When Chuck spoke of an "aha!" moment, he meant something like the flash of strategic clarity that shores up the vitality of the intellect.

Chuck was searching for the solution to a riddle; therapy, by contrast, often asks us to remain with problems that cannot be solved in that way at all. And so I dismissed this idea a bit hastily, as a flip, an easy detour, replacing the game I preferred: the gradual recognition of emotional desires versus fears, and the conflicts arising between them. This oversight led to the thorny moment I will describe.

I was around this time acclimating to therapeutic work, having recently ended my stint as a rehab counselor for substance abuse. I hastily framed his *aha!* seeking as a demand on himself, and on me implicitly, for a shortcut.

Here was familiar pressure, as with the recovering patients I so often counseled, to "get this solved and move on with life." But what needed to be solved were longstanding existential dilemmas, and their articulation.

Thus I heard Chuck's call for insight as familiar, another gifted individual over-relying on intellect to "solve" deeply emotional, personalized problems, even as said intellect had often rationalized drinking. (If all you have is a hammer ….)

What I heard, in other words, was another version of my own alcoholic father. (And Chuck once sheepishly informed he often had "a cocktail or two, or three" after especially tense days—a topic we curiously did not return to.)

I recall a specific moment with Chuck, now tinged with slight regret on my part. He occasionally cracked wise about my office size and other patients in the waiting room, usually followed by a blushing apology and a reminder he could be a bit of a jerk. (I had nothing to add after hearing the latter.)

One day he mentioned a surprise phone call from his loathed rival, who phoned for advice on a thorny corporate matter. Pride got the better of Chuck; he had a good solution and would have been happy to consult, for a fee. "But I'm not a beggar," he said, a bit haughtily, and told his caller he had nothing to offer, and hung up. He quietly said, "Maybe that was a mistake."

I asked if he had feelings about not offering a proposal, given his financial strain (with one child completing college, another starting soon).

He surprised me by saying, with a semi-sneer, "Oh, you're asking about *feelings*. Geez I feel like a *girl* …" Noting my surprise, he pivoted to another subject. (So hard for him to not be the boss.)

For a moment the room seemed to fill with the humiliation he was trying to push away. I felt it too—a bit stung, and momentarily off-balance. What the devil was going on?

In Chuck's world, the reader has probably surmised, discussing feelings belonged to a different game or grammar (Wittgenstein, 2009)[1], a foreign language best left to others (perhaps females). Strategy, negotiation, and insight were signs of potency, whereas reflecting on and from within emotion signaled defeat: a kind of grammatical emasculation.

Chuck's father, I learned early on, had been a military captain. Chuck's "like a girl" remark was not simply bravado or misogyny but a protest against the humiliating shift from solving problems to being conquered by them, his father (one imagines) smirking from the sidelines. Chuck had never been granted the more intimate grammar of asking for help; instead the binaries prevailed: you either had answers or you didn't, had the smarts or went home early.

Even coming to therapy might have been like crying "uncle" for Chuck: a humiliation. I wish I had responded with the empathic observance that some part of him surely must have hated being there. Given the paternalistic pressures just described, it made sense. The sneering I heard—toward feelings, my office, the sad-looking "shlubs" in the waiting room—had been echoing all along. His was a one-up or one-down world, and his presence on the couch tilted toward degradation.

He had sounded, in his telling, hurt and humiliated at his ouster (including a chintzy severance package). Now, on top of that, he was being asked to feel things ("like a girl") while needing the consultation of a guy who would not provide the Hollywood breakthrough moment—complete with orchestral strings—that he hoped would get him back in the fight. (He strongly disliked or even hated, I suspected, not being the boss, which seemed to cause conflict at home.)

He also, I imagined, yearned to be stronger than his critical father, whose Oedipal control and success (living comfortably on a pension) was probably hard to swallow. In a way, he implicitly hoped *I* would now swallow such bile, a telling communication. (Which also told me something about his style, the sarcasm that alienated others.)

At the time, however, I was so taken aback that I did not know what to say. Most of my greatest interventions are delivered in the rear-view mirror, or the chapters of a book.

Easy to be smart in hindsight. And equating intellect with potency is a common illusion crushed repeatedly by life—like Sisyphus's rock. Such crushing actually communicated loudest of all. Chuck had suffered a death to his self-image in being thrown out of his company, giving his father a chance to subtly gloat and remind his son he never liked the company to begin with. (And how about that lunch?)

I often think of Camus' line that we must imagine Sisyphus happy; if so, then Sisyphus does not overthink it: he *acts,* embracing his task and situation as fully as possible. Longing for the mental power to sidestep angst, an aspect of our mortal vulnerability, is delusion, not action. The fantasy that a sufficiently brilliant insight could dissolve absurdity mistakes existential struggle for a solvable riddle. Therapy often begins precisely where that expectation collapses.

Chuck's "like a girl" comment also echoed my father's hollow bravado, and baited me into thinking Chuck held no truck with discussing emotion. I heard his statement as contempt, ignoring the background terror.

Chuck was clearly stuck in quicksand, with no name for it and no way to grasp its deeper meaning, desperate for the rescuing vine he had always managed to find on his own. Even his wife had functioned largely as a mirror of his success rather than a dialogic ally. Now that vine took the form of his therapist's outstretched hand; though dependence, in his world, was for sissies, having been burned by his father and now by his rival. What he failed to see—along with his therapist, come to think of it—was that I was right there with him in the muck!

But he disliked being there, and distrusted or even resented me (the one who *knew* while he didn't), especially since—as with his father, colleague, and wife—he needed me.

Therapy dwells in the irrational, the fallout of a human existence fraught with surprisingly cruel twists, testing our character in difficult ways. Each treatment, too, has such moments, if we are lucky. Chuck had come seeking the right insight, the key that would unlock the problem. Yet the work gradually revealed something else: not a solution to a riddle, but the slow reshaping of the grammar of the riddle itself. By this I mean those shifting forms of life, through which his experience could be *acknowledged* rather than shoehorned into an enigmatic test question.

It is also human to dread these "life lessons" life foists upon us, quite without our permission. The Greeks understood this, as Camus (1983) also recognized in his discussion of Sisyphus, and our existential upending. Still we try, nowadays especially, to rewrite the algorithm, bypass tragedy like technical snafus awaiting a system update. Chuck came to therapy hoping for such a cheat code, a flash of brilliance that would restore his footing, the thrill of isolated thought.

Therapy more often resembles Sisyphus' labor: returning again and again to the stone before us, which for the longest stretches does not seem to budge. If we imagine Sisyphus happy, it may be because he accepts the task itself, including the strange relief of its impossibility. Therapy at its best may help us do the same.

Note

1 See my introduction for an explanation of what Wittgenstein meant by *grammar.*

References

Camus, A. (1983). *The myth of Sisyphus* (J. O'Brien, Trans.) Vintage International. Originally published 1955.

Stolorow, R. (2007). *Trauma and human existence*. Routledge.

Wittgenstein, L. (2009). *Philosophical investigations* (4th ed.) (G.E.M. Anscombe, P.M.S. Hacker, & J. Schulte, Trans.) (P.M.S. Hacker, & J. Schulte, Eds.) Blackwell Publishing Ltd. Originally published 1953.

7 Certainty and Its Discontents

Words Apart

Part 1

Recovery culture often relies on slogans that promise clarity and relief from emotional uncertainty. Such phrases can inspire, but they can also function defensively, warding off affects that resist easy expression. Therapists are not immune to this pull. Patient and analyst alike can become caught in a search for the "right words": phrases that sound wise or therapeutic yet fail to "move the ball," in addressing deeper relational dilemmas.

Often in early stages I am called upon to bolster rather than examine the pet phrases patients borrow from recovery programs, self-help books, or other sources—as if isolated phrases might conjure the togetherness longed for, an end to long-term confinement. (But then, who is the jailer?)

A parallel process occurs with therapists in *their* attachment to theory or favored concepts. The following vignette illustrates how both parties became caught up in a search for magical words, language that sounded polished and wise, yet accomplished little.

Sarah, an attractive, creative patient in her early forties, was sober from alcohol and marijuana. She sought my help for what she called her "codependency": men who were charming at first, promising the world, until their behavior painfully upended the sales pitch. *Why am I such an easy mark*, she bemoaned.

I made the error of thinking I might rebalance this conundrum by sounding empathic, as if it were a matter of "sounding" helpful, thus soothing her troubled soul. Here, I secretly hoped, was a man who would genuinely see and hear Sarah, for the first time perhaps, in line with the ideals of relational therapy (as I understood it): the provision of a safe haven that might unblock the path to fulfillment.

In other words, I misunderstood completely.

"Codependence" is not my favorite term but one Sarah found helpful. It spoke to her of her own unworthiness, since *she* was stupid enough to depend upon such losers. Such judgment locked her out of her own psyche, unable to understand her strivings—a latchkey kid without the key.

DOI: 10.4324/9781003598534-7

Sarah seemed to expect miracles from compromised men. What went missing in her musings were the dynamics driving these romantic implosions, how she remained so "inept" (her word)—or really, un-practiced—in negotiating or understanding her own needs and red lines of others' behavior. Such needs were met or not met, men "got it" or they didn't, the relationship a home run or a forfeit, due to lack of interest. Sarah herself carried subtle demands for the certainty of outcomes, struggling with a fear that she said was "dumb," "unnecessary," or "a turn-off."

Her early life was a blizzard of abandonment, where accommodating her misattuned, often narcissistic father, Bill, was a survivalist must. She learned that what she had to say didn't really matter; never taken in, taken seriously, or heard at all. (In this way an environment confers—or dismisses—the value of the child's words.)

Bill was not her biological father, but the partner of Sarah's mother when Sarah was born. Sarah's biological father had disappeared long before. When Sarah was eight or nine her mother disappeared for almost a year, an addict/alcoholic and rock groupie (the glorious seventies), often hospitalized for delusions, depression, or medical problems related to drinking.

Sarah recalled receiving anguished calls from her hospitalized mother, begging for a visit. Teenage Sarah would reluctantly acquiesce, met not with warmth but venomous criticism for staying away so long, which only fed the aloofness that led to her condemnation. (She could not win for losing.)

Meanwhile Bill, the man she called dad, adopted Sarah out of pity and obligation, as he reminded her throughout her upbringing. Bill often implied she "owed him" fealty, in the form of constant praise. Sarah became his confidante, listening uneasily to his romantic woes and quiet contempt for the female love he both needed and demanded, such uneasiness quelled in adolescence via her use of marijuana. Pot, in other words, became *her* caregiver.

"I just didn't want to be there," she said of these endless "chats." Later the thrill of pot, romance, and sex proved a corrective to inner dullness, even if short lived; abandonment became the built-in price of such thrill rides. ("Mary Jane" at least was loyal.)

Sarah was taught that her role, the cost of her security, was to idealize and shore up a man's worthiness. This undermined her own ability to speak and think reliably of her own strivings and fears: chattel to systemic *angst.* Such an arrangement became an enslavement she loathed but could not escape (again stuck in the tower). She longed to be more genuine, but what did that mean or sound like?

This reflects the contextual nature of words. There is no essence of "genuineness" outside of specific actions and situations. As Wittgenstein (2009) wrote, any inner process "stands in need of outward criteria" (§ 580): tone of voice, facial expression, gesture, and speech.

"Inner" is also of course a convention, tempting literalism at times. When emotion cannot learn to speak, frictions nonetheless remain, the body their interpreter—amplifying the temptation of pot, alcohol, and so on.

Sarah lacked any map of her inner life, drawn with attunement, as any such sketching was hastily erased by Bill's ramblings and mother's criticisms; such a map always led to the needs of the other.

"Genuine" anguish and isolation, then, were relieved via others' stabilizing speech; this was the familiar balm, the "codependency" she hated and could not do without. She spoke of "freedom" without knowing what it might sound or feel like, beyond a grunt of incomprehension, or fear. Could someone, anyone, please fill her in?

Keenly intelligent, she sought self-help phrases or other concepts to unlock this solitary confinement, to get her down from the tower. When stoned, smokers often think it is the musings and not the narcotizing background that leads to "cool thoughts." She now seemed to hope, with the help of her trusty therapist, that she would learn to mentally grasp a man's inner character, all at once preferably, in order to determine if the light was green or red (yes or no). Her therapist might offer such "tools," as he himself was male.

In other words, here again the other had the last word.

The men Sarah chose, even those sober in recovery, often turned out to have problems with money, career, and/or compulsive porn use, despite their initial pizzazz. She said, "How did my picker get so broken?" Here I longed for the perfect recovery-type slogan, and came up silent.

She hated herself for having sex too soon, before allowing for real assessment (I had cautioned her to wait)—but what if she waited too long, and he bolted? Was she destined for loneliness, like her mother? "He seems put together," she said about a new prospect, hypnotically charismatic (and possibly, I feared, a player). She watched me after saying this, as if waiting for a thumbs-up or down. "One date at a time," I said, smiling benignly. In no time she reported her infatuation.

I observed flashes of irritation or wariness (toward me or her dates?) that she quickly sidestepped. "No guy wants an angry woman," she said, after I encouraged her to vent her frustration with the now-vanished suitor; she had decided the light was green, and after a few romantic, sex-filled weekends, he confessed he was still in love with his ex-girlfriend.

She often expressed wariness of her own rage; I responded, a bit hurriedly, of the hurt "beneath" such fire, a soothing detour for therapists uneasy with rawer affect, a concept of convenience: a common myth we tell ourselves. How can anything lie "beneath" an anger or rage *itself never recognized*? In saying this we risk the pretense of omniscience, or X-ray vision.

After yet another relationship fizzled out—"but he promised he'd stick around," she lamented—Sarah asked me point-blank, with edgy impatience, what needed to change *in her*, to avoid dating more schmucks, as if I had a magic spell under my chair. "Where am I going wrong, what's my problem, no more bullshitting," she said.

I felt like I was on a game show. She sat there, watching and waiting.

I was clearly on the spot, vaguely resenting the question, while empathically understanding *why* she asked. (Who doesn't want their money's worth?)

But we could not seem to ever get to that why, lacking any guidelines or means of discussion, all of it projected onto the chess board of dating, the was-he-or-wasn't-he the one. It was like visiting Paris without a map; one could see the Eiffel Tower, without ever getting there.

I had privately wondered about her long-term reluctance in confronting or at least inquiring about her partners' ongoing (excuse me) bullshit, along with reluctance to follow any of the suggestions she asked for from me. Any caution I advised was practically a dog-whistle for a weekend tryst, sooner rather than later. Perhaps romantic toil was a distraction, given the unresolved chaos in her life—dealing with her self-absorbed dad, harsh sponsor, outbursts from mom (still), work and financial stress—that we had yet to discuss.

Well ok, fine, but I still had no idea what to say to Sarah, our session nearly over….

Then I remembered something. A week or two beforehand, Sarah mentioned she was tired of her dates (and dad) "mansplaining" things they clearly knew nothing about. She said it would be far better if a guy just said, "I don't know," rather than arrogantly wing it.

And so I now said, gently but with confidence it would work, "I don't know …."

She exploded.

"Oh that's great," she said, jaw clenched, face bleached with rage, "nobody knows, no one ever knows a fuckin' thing. I'm sick of 'I don't know.' When is *someone gonna know*?" She pounded the armrest with her fist.

I was stunned, as if in free fall, my feet having plunged through the floorboards.

But, I protested silently, *this is what you asked for!*

Then I noticed the humiliation and hurt on her face … the familiar self-loathing creeping in … as if her feet were *always* crashing through floorboards, because she again was stupidly not paying enough attention, had trusted yet another disappointing male.

"It's like I'm never allowed to ask for things," she said, tearing up.

This … is what we were avoiding.

Not so much the rage, but the inevitable disappointment, the shame of the annihilated need, humiliation at its return.

I encouraged her to share more of her reaction. She hesitated, then said she felt shrugged off, dismissed, that I had spoken with a smirk. I asked, "Like, 'why are you asking such a dumb question'?" She nodded. I winced.

My error became apparent: she was looking for close attunement and male strength, not merely the right words.

Perhaps this is why she both clung to *and vaguely resented* the slogans: a life raft that (again) failed her, even though she was a "good girl" in recovery. Resentment is discussed as toxic to sobriety in recovery; perhaps we had both shied away from it, until she (fortunately) insisted on speaking up, and out.

I told Sarah I imagined my response was glib, and I was sorry for that. I added that I felt a bit on the spot, as any answer here was complex, and far from black and white, no handy bullet point, though this might well sound like hedging, a dodge, even … disappointing to her: yet another man failing to meet the moment, which I was loath to do.

She softened. "Oh. Why didn't you just say *that*?"

Great question.

I said that I was sensitive to language, sometimes overthinking it, and had perhaps pressured *myself* to know, in just the right way. Maybe I avoided stepping her on her toes, as she avoided stepping on "his" (the man of the moment).

I wanted to answer. But what was needed here was collaborative cartography: a map of where she was and where she might want to go.

She asked, with anxious rapidity, "Ok but *how do we do that I don't know how*?"

I said, with deliberate slowness, that we might start with talking about how scary it was to need or want something from a man, including me. Her question was a plea for getting it right: *am I a fool for wanting?* But the language game of yes/no was itself at issue; we needed to expand, to break through the walls like a remodeling project.

In this way we might have space to discuss the despair and terror behind the question, the terror of her need, in light of such profound neglect.

"Profound neglect," she repeated. "I never heard that before."

But she had *lived it*. Perhaps genuineness is a means of speaking what the body already knows but is too frightened to say. Starting with this fear of speaking—of getting it wrong, saying it incorrectly (meaning one shouldn't have said it at all)—can get dialogue rolling.

A few minutes later she quietly remarked, "I just feel so alone all the time."

I waited a few moments…then wondered aloud if finding a male attracted to her was redemptive, proof that she was worthy, undeserving of her mother's criticisms and dad's narcissism, which otherwise served as proof, that stark imprisonment in the tower.

She nodded, reached for a Kleenex.

She said, while walking to the door, "Guess I need to keep coming back."

She didn't.

Part 2

After another two or three sessions, Sarah texted me to say she was "taking a break" from treatment and hiring a dating coach.

The discussion I insisted on didn't get us far; she merely assured me that, in so many words, *it's not you, it's me*.

I recalled my doctoral advisor telling me that, for some patients, the first firm boundary they ever set is with their analyst. Sarah stuck with her plan.

What had I missed? I had tried to help her get comfortable with uncertainty, perhaps too quickly. Sarah never seemed to imagine she could be the one saying no, until she said exactly that to her treatment.

Perhaps I had been swayed by my own desire for "progress," hoping to reach the tortured child-self that no one, including Sarah, quite wanted to acknowledge: the child under the bed while caregivers argued … the door-slam of her mother leaving the house—for the night, then for good. At least now the slamming was in her control.

Perhaps it was difficult for her to take me in; non-physical contact may have felt unpersuasive, since no empathic reflection (no matter how accurate)—especially at once a week—can *on its own* dispel dread or despair. There may also have been humiliation after her outburst, or difficulty tolerating the presence of a receptive male, with a wish for literal holding rather than skinless empathy.

Perhaps perhaps ….

I recalled I had been one of a long line of therapists. Her staying nearly two years—her longest stretch—was a victory, of sorts. She had at least finally found permission to desire, to want, with a little less shame.

In fact she emailed me a few months later, to say she was dating an older man with whom she had really connected, informing me—not without pride—that she was able to inform him of his bothersome habits (news-scrolling in bed); he appeared receptive to the feedback. "It's all going well," she said, "so now I'll really need you, lol!" (I haven't heard from her since.)

There was so much of Sarah's forgotten history, aspects of a tragedy untold (and *unnoticed*). It is easy to overlook, especially early in our careers, the impact of our presence, of a patient simply *there* with us. (What constitutes such "there" for them? What in the world do they think of us, really?)

Such presence awakens both desire and dread, partly because longing is so difficult to express under the best of circumstances. And patients usually show up feeling at their worst.

Meanwhile clinicians seek to hear the pain "beneath" defenses. Yet there is no beneath, only attempts to explore its possibility through the presence of inner life, or its wary absence. Often we *co-create* the "inner," the practice of psychological language games, co-establishing new practices. Both need to have grammatical skin in the game—lean in, take risks—where words come to symbolize the touch of skinless contact.

Any and all theory is but a beginning.

At least Sarah left without any retaliation or attack, with the genuine promise of an open door should she wish to return; perhaps she needed to know it was permitted, having found the father she needed, one she could finally leave at home.

Reference

Wittgenstein, L. (2009). *Philosophical investigations* (4th ed.) (G.E.M. Anscombe, P.M.S. Hacker, & J. Schulte, Trans.) (P.M.S. Hacker, & J. Schulte, Eds.) Blackwell Publishing Ltd. Originally published 1953.

8 Living Speech and Analytic Silence

Playing Dead

Sometimes we are tempted to fill the silence, rather than listen to what it seems to say.

The impulse to speak can be especially strong when a patient's certainties preempt exploration, narrowing the rules of the language game. In such moments we may use words as placeholders, as if keeping space for ourselves in the face of foreclosing utterances.

"I'm a failure," Robby liked to say, "no doubt about it." There was something constraining about these statements, repeated blandly, like a weather report.

To me they felt like the strain of an undersized shirt collar; I disliked their either/or quality. "Sounds like your inner critic," I might say, to which he would nod affably, then fall silent. A pensive quiet took hold; soon we were both stuck. *What are we doing here,* I wondered.

Robby was an attorney in his early thirties, with a pleasant demeanor and eagerness to start. He wanted help, ostensibly, in curbing his compulsive use of porn and "cam girls," models who enacted online fantasies for ten dollars a minute. "What kind of loser does this stuff?" he said (apparently, he did).

Now he sought reinvention, tired of his solitary confinement and pathetic habits. Yet he feared "real women," as he put it, becoming tongue-tied on dates, trying too hard to be funny, fearful of sounding "stupid."

This to my ears sounded more benevolent than his self-disgust; charming were his hopes to impress, scenes from a romantic comedy. But for Robby this was more of a legal drama, where everyone—including his therapist—came fitted in judicial robes.

It was a part I refused, kindly and repeatedly questioning the stubborn vetoing of his own character. But such veto of the veto was a foreclosure of another kind. I heard the rigidity of his statements as *the problem,* without understanding its utility as a solution (as something to lean on perhaps, preventing collapse).

Still, it bothered me.

Robby knew even as a boy that he would grow up to become a lawyer—just like his father, a fearsome litigator who could be friendly with colleagues

DOI: 10.4324/9781003598534-8

yet intimidating at home. Young Robby yearned for his dad's approval, always just out of reach. He settled for the consolation prize of compliance, staying silent at his father's side, parroting his opinions, annoying his mother, who would turn away muttering, "like father, like son."

His father liked to sit after dinner with his gin and tonics, watching news channels and critiquing everything as "dumb," barbed eviscerations of the witless, which included just about everyone (except himself). Folded into the cut were Robby's sister and (especially) his mother, often the butt of his father's crude humor. (It sounded like they detested each other.) Robby felt guilty for not defending his mother, staying silent, lest the verbal scalpel come for him.

His mother, of Slavic origin, still struggled with English at times, her malapropisms evoking her husband's gin-tinged bemusement or mockery, prompting her to sullenly withdraw. This added to Robby's conviction that *his* words had to be surgically precise. He also felt ashamed of not defending her. It was unclear if she ever sensed or responded to this extinguishing guilt (no wonder that the distance of virtual sex, later in adulthood, remained alluring).

"That's a big responsibility," I once said. He shrugged, "It is what it is."

He filled in more of his backstory, where after a relatively happy upbringing (really?), he became more withdrawn in adolescence, afraid of girls and anything less than straight A's. He was terrified of any imperfection, studying until dawn, exhausted by test-time, leading to the low grades he feared. Verbal eviscerations followed. Such perfectionism dogged him in college, where assignments were late and he gradually fell behind.

This led to a period of sagging grades and depression, although he "snapped out of it" on his own, he said (proudly?) Soon he was devoting himself to law school, passing the bar, and landing at a firm specializing in copyrights. His salary was more than ample, though his father grumbled that his son had not followed in his litigator's footsteps. "I'm just not cut out for it," he sighed, another strike against him.

Once I observed that he sounded skilled at his job, that his bosses seemed to like him. He demurred; he had a photographic memory, and the work was not difficult. If only he had the stomach for courtroom battles, like dad.

Sometimes he told me of his plans to improve his life: take an acting class, join Toastmasters … like moving pieces on a board. Such moves seemed good enough, as if statements alone did the trick. (Later, of course, he dinged himself for a lack of follow-up, as if realizing that any happiness found there would be ephemeral.)

Law was a fairly good metaphor for how he lived: managing indefinite experience through definite concepts. This included the cam girl activity, measured out in dollars and minutes; the price built into the interaction, bypassing the negotiation needed in "real" relationships (whatever that meant). He was even prompt in paying me, ended sessions *on the dot*—leaving hurriedly, as if he had taken enough of my time.

The psychic costs to him were harder to measure, unmentioned as they were in the statutes inscribed in paternal handwriting, enacted with the comfort of perfunctory duty.

I wanted to amend the constitution here, yet lacked a majority.

There were times when Robby would pause over a troubling interaction and say, "I wonder why this bothers me so much", as if it should not.

I would respond here, in the spirit of support, offering possible answers: *well, it sounds difficult, they really pissed you off, maybe you're not allowed to have feelings*—to which he would again nod, not saying much, looking pensive or confused … as if I had spoken Swahili.

Our impasse was not only clinical but *grammatical*, in Wittgenstein's (2009) sense of the term: the unspoken "rules" or customs governing what counts as meaningful speech. But silences too can speak, once we attune to their distinctiveness. (Anxiety makes excellent earplugs.)

After hearing a patient's self-flagellations, the analyst's impulse may be to respond rather than wait—to interpret, reassure, or elaborate, to keep the conversation moving. Yet these responses can unwittingly echo the same "rules" governing the patient's speech, a swapping out of certainties (new wine in old bottles).

Withstanding silence, by contrast, can interrupt the expected sequence of conversational moves. When the anticipated response does not arrive, the language game is briefly thrown off rhythm, creating a small opening: a tension that calls for patience. I often moved to diffuse this tension, too quickly, restoring our systemic *staccato.*

The hermeneutical value of my inquiries stood in tension with Robby's utterances. But many struggling with compulsivity cannot recognize or make use of reflective space, for what counts as *personally* significant. (And even practiced musicians need time to learn new songs.) I often forgot Robby was a beginner—as was I, in knowing Robby.

Both Wittgenstein and Lacan were preoccupied with the forms of language that shape what can intelligibly be said. Each explored, from different angles, how speech can authorize *and* imprison the subject within a particular grammar.

Lacan spent his life examining our embeddedness in the structures of language. He describes language as a symbolic order into which we are born: already positioned within it, even as we babble our first words. The mobility of that order depends upon whether speech can move beyond inherited certainties, allowing new meanings—and new positions for the speaker—to emerge. When such movement becomes restricted, speech may harden into repetitive formulations that function less as expressions than as rules governing what can be said.

In Robby's case, this rigidity ensnared me as well, inviting responses that matched (rather than loosened) his certainties.

We might instead ask, what is the function of certainties such as Robby's? What position do they occupy, and what move are they making in what kind of game? The lack of possible answers may be the loudest silence of all.

Let us not understand this too quickly.

Part of the challenge here is the slipperiness of speech. The word person itself belongs to the symbolic order; it already holds a position. In suffocating environments like Robby's, *personhood* is cast in the chilling shadow of caregivers, draining the life from subjective speech. A cigar is just a cigar, and Robby was his father's son. (The end.)

Early misattunement, in such scenarios, represents not the injury the analyst so clearly sees—but the "failure" of the patient to overlook its constriction, its enforced purpose as a sign saying "stop" or "detour." *What* is detoured remains unrecognized and unimportant.

But there is another way of hearing statements such as, "I'm a failure." True, yes, but not as intended. He had "failed" a task I viewed as impossible: to speak individually *in a system foreclosing such possibility*, to speak like a subject (as Lacan might say) while smothered by objectifying demands.

These unspeakable (and painful) experiences are the gold we hope to mine. For Robby such metal was closer to plutonium; it threatened the expected order.

Robby in fact often experienced my curiosity as another demand: to *demonstrate* interest and cooperation. The result is what Lacan (2001) called *empty speech,* a hollowing out of selfhood. Such speech circles subjectivity like the outer ring of a wheel, leaving a void in the middle. The familiar role of "good patient" rescues them from the most impossible task of all: speaking for themselves.

Agentic centering remains exiled, expansiveness is criminal, as it might acknowledge a subjectivity strangled in its crib (with caregivers the prime suspects). Analysis comes to resemble a crime scene: the chalk outline of the missing patient. But we alone notice the silhouette.

Thus the rigidifying impact of Robby's certitudes. He could not yet recognize any alternative register. I myself heard overtones of tragedy.

Lacan (2001) suggests that the child's first words—*mama* or *dada*—name not only the parent but also an absence that makes the naming necessary. Language replaces what is missing in the gap that facilitates speech.

Language never fully fills this gap. We are always encountering a limit. Here a kind of improvisation is needed, a "riffing" beyond the repetitive rhythms.

But early systems such as Robby's deny this limit, imposing peremptory commands that foreclose language's expansion.

Is this why Robby's flailing attempts at romance were so flatly described (the equanimity of failure)? He often said he had no idea what to talk about on dates (as in session, often enough), that small talk bored him; meantime he tried too hard to be funny, asked personal questions too soon or "over-shared," lost in meandering monologues … though he always picked up the check, as men are obliged to do.

I inwardly winced upon hearing all this, him splashing about in the deep. "Dating isn't easy," I would say, "for anyone."

"It shouldn't be this hard," he once replied.

He then confessed, as if underlining the point, to hiring a cam girl—one of his "regulars"—after another bad date. This regular was paid to denigrate him with obscenities while he masturbated on camera; this was somehow easier than talking to a real person. (Yet the real obscenity, to my mind, was ever unnamed.)

He described to me how he would sit, afterward, staring vacantly at the blank screen, the pathetic isolation of his life. (Here he was having his cake and choking on it too.)

I thanked him for telling me, gently said, "We can talk more about it if you want." He didn't; the verdict was already in.

Then he found a gal with whom he got on well. Was this progress? Wendy sounded interesting and seemed to like him. They had a few enjoyable dates, despite his mild ambivalence, though when it came time for sex he found he could not "last." Wendy cautiously (perhaps anxiously) suggested Viagra; Robby withdrew, sullen and humiliated. He stopped returning her calls; she ended it with an email saying she hated being ghosted.

I too felt deflated hearing this, and for the first time empathized with the other in the equation. Every date had been a *fait accompli,* including his regulars with me, all confirming the "loser" verdict delivered long ago: case closed. Nothing could shake this bone from his bite.

I felt out of ideas, suggestions, or inspiration. The clinical air was thick, pressing down (I sensed) on both of us. Perhaps we needed some clinical Viagra. *How long*, I asked myself, *before he bails on me too*. The acrid whiff of failure wafted through; perhaps he *wanted* us to fail, to preserve the status quo. *If so,* I thought, *then fine, good luck and godspeed.*

But in sitting there, saying nothing, I noticed my own anxiety, which had likely spurred so many of my statements, these cash-free giveaways, as if to enliven the proceedings, counter the deadening spell. But who or what felt dead, and did *this* serve a purpose beyond the indifference I sometimes envisioned? I had vaguely organized this as resistance, a kind of opposition. Was it?

I waited, and after a few awkward, long moments, Robby asked if I had any thoughts.

"Not really," I said. "That is, I'm … not sure what to say."

Robby chewed on his lip, concerned. "I'm probably a difficult patient."

"Actually," I said, "I wish you were *more* difficult." He was surprised by this and asked what I meant.

I said, "Well, when you say something like 'I'm a failure' or 'I'm stupid,' it's like the end of the story. There's nothing more to it."

"But it's not what I want!" he said, sitting up.

I asked him, myself surprised, what it might be that he wanted. He watched me silently, as if confused.

I recalled just then a moment early in my own analysis. Just after getting married, I expressed to my analyst my fondness for my new father-in-law. My analyst asked what kind of relationship I might want with him, given my own longings for paternal oversight and affection.

I fell silent, unsure how to answer, and felt ashamed for not having the words, thinking, *It's not a hard question, genius.* But it was, because it did not occur to me that I might have a say in such things. It was like viewing a map of an unknown city, and being asked to name its neighborhoods.

Was it possible that Robby felt compelled to provide such names *with certainty,* despite a muddied map, the only *safe* answer being his loser-dom? I had also asked him, upon his first arrival, *So what do you think the problem is?* Perhaps "I'm a loser" was the only reliable fall-back; better than having nothing to say.

Robby struggled (as I had) to say what he wanted. Was it because any inscription of the "rules" had never been up to him? "Robby" as such had yet to exist. In saying "you" I was addressing an absence, a ghost chained to repetition; the room itself felt haunted.

I gently said, "It's hard to say what you want." He nodded.

I recalled his telling me that his father, in earlier days, would grill him with questions about his schoolwork. "What happened if you got it wrong?" I once asked. "There was no 'wrong'," he said.

Which meant that, if he answered that question—*what do you want*—he had *better be right.* But the only certainty possible in that case was his current stuckness. Thus the circle repeated: the emptiness of speech. Ever signified was his remaining at his father's side; to go beyond that was to wade into frightfully powerful currents.

So often I felt immobilized by his staying ankle-deep; it had never occurred to me to ask if he knew how to swim.

I then, shortly after this session, remembered a moment that did not register at the time. This was yet another of my comments about the inner critic that seemed to shut him down. "You're probably right," he said, murmuring, "and you said it much better than I could."

How could I have let this slip by?

This meant he had already flunked, as in his freshman year in college: days and nights of staring at the ceiling, choking on despair, self-hatred, and a loneliness too painful and shameful to name.

There was another angle to all this: my own anxieties, cluttering the field of play. I grew up with an alcoholic father who enforced a game similar to Robby's, with inflexible demands for answers. To not have them was fatal; my father liked to grill me on what he had just said, a demand to parrot his insights, likely sensing my waning interest (go figure) in his monologues. I became an annex for his need, my name a reflection of the stature he enforced.

This implicated me in my *pas de deux* with Robby; urgent it seemed, to demonstrate (perform?) my beneficence as the anti-dad. *You're free here,* I wanted to tell him, *and safe. I'm neither your father nor mine; I left that game long ago.*

Perhaps we were both treading water, amidst currents we could not yet trust.

Yet a subtle shift occurred when I asked about the wants he was not sure deserved "airtime," even internally. He remarked in a moment of candor, clearly embarrassed, that he had not felt all that attracted to Wendy—but felt he "ought" to keep seeing her, because she liked him. "And I know you think I should be dating," he added.

He was not wrong. I hoped for him to be less lonely; but the key to such novel interaction lay between us, in the room rather than in the world.

No wonder that, with me, he repeated his mantra of failure. Hearing such unspoken suffering ratchets up the pressure; external changes seem to promise relief. But the patient may then believe more "straight-A's" are expected of them, distracting from the problem hiding in plain sight.

Robby was in a way protecting me, saying he did not know the rules of the dating I encouraged, the spoken desire I strained to hear; he would probably screw it up, so *don't go investing in me, you'll be disappointed too.*

He mentioned to me one day that his father, now elderly, aging and weak, had been hinting at a forgiveness he hoped his son might deliver. (His parents were long divorced, his mother pretty much out of the picture.) Forgiveness feels expensive when the debt of recognition remains unpaid. His father had never really "owned" the psychic straitjacketing of his son. Still Robby felt he ought to forgive, another square to land one's piece upon.

After a long pause, I asked Robby what he was thinking. He said, "Well part of me wants to forgive, and the other part …."

I waited.

He sighed. "Well I'd like to ask why he drank like a fish and was such an asshole to my mom." He paused. "Maybe that's harsh."

"Yes," I said, "you better take that back *right now.*" I playfully wagged a finger at him.

He paused, then erupted with laughter. Suddenly, he was *there.*

References

Lacan, J. (2001). *Ecrits: A selection.* (A. Sheridan, Trans.) Routledge Classics. Originally published 1977.

Wittgenstein, L. (2009). *Philosophical investigations* (4th ed.) (G.E.M. Anscombe, P.M.S. Hacker, & J. Schulte, Trans.) (P.M.S. Hacker, & J. Schulte, Eds.) Blackwell Publishing Ltd. Originally published 1953.

Index

Note: Page numbers followed by 'n' refer to notes.

For Product Safety Concerns and Information please contact our EU representative GPSR@taylorandfrancis.com
Taylor & Francis Verlag GmbH, Kaufingerstraße 24, 80331 München, Germany

www.ingramcontent.com/pod-product-compliance
Lightning Source LLC
LaVergne TN
LVHW020654100826
845148LV00012B/2488

* 9 7 8 1 0 3 2 9 8 0 6 1 4 *